Ditch the Script

Get Everything You Need from the Client for Successful Hypnotherapy and Set Up to Wrap Up with Results

Wendie Webber

TribeofHealers.com

Ditch the Script: Get Everything You Need from the Client for Successful Hypnotherapy and Set Up to Wrap Up with Results

Wendie Webber

Copyright © 2021 Wendie Webber
All Rights Reserved.

All rights reserved. No part of this publication may be reproduced, distributed, or transmitted in any form or by any means, including photocopying, recording, or other electronic or mechanical methods without the prior written permission from the author, except in the case of brief quotations embodied in critical reviews and certain non-commercial uses permitted by copyright law.

The information given in this book should not be treated as a substitute for professional medical advice; always consult a medical practitioner. Any use of information in this book is at the reader's discretion and risk. Neither the author nor the publisher can be held responsible for any loss, claim, or damage arising out of the use, or misuse, of the suggestions made, the failure to take medical advice, or for any material on third-party websites.

ISBN Print Book: 978-1-7774121-2-8

Wendie Webber
Address: PO Box 55027 SOUTHGATE MALL PO
Nanaimo, British Columbia, Canada

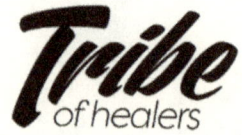

www.TribeofHealers.com

TABLE OF CONTENTS

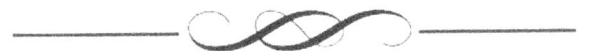

TABLE OF CONTENTS i
WHY READ THIS BOOK i
WHAT OTHERS SAY iii
CHAPTER 1: Success is in Your Set Up 1
CHAPTER 2: Qualify Your Clients 9
CHAPTER 3: Critical Qualifying Questions 17
CHAPTER 4: Take a History 27
CHAPTER 5: Intake Assessments 45
CHAPTER 6: Symptom Resolution Keys 53
CHAPTER 7: Set Up to Wrap Up 79
CHAPTER 8: Set Up for Forgiveness Work 95
CHAPTER 9: Ditch the Script 99
CHAPTER 10: Set Up for the Next Session 111
CHAPTER 11: Conclusion 117
Ready to learn more? 120
Wendie Webber 121
Get Ready for Regression! 122

My heartfelt thanks to my angel, Susanne Neuenschwander, for her loving support and diligence in translating The Devil's Therapy into German.

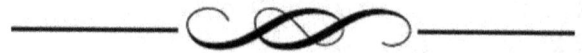

WHY READ THIS BOOK

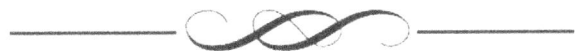

The front door was wide open and Mom was nowhere in sight.

I stood there, at the top of the stairs of my family's two-story house, realizing that there was a whole world waiting to be explored—at the bottom of those stairs! And, I stepped forward, tumbling down those stairs.

That first step was a real doozie. At the tender age of eighteen months, I learned an important lesson that day.

"Just do it!" isn't always your best strategy.

You probably know this. "Just do it!" was an iconic slogan created by the sports apparel company Nike. These three magic words quickly became a cultural meme. But did you know that the phrase was inspired by the final words of a notorious murderer? It's true. Just before being executed by firing squad, serial killer Gary Gilmore was quoted as saying, "Let's do this!"

If you happen to be a gung-ho, damn-the-torpedoes type of person, "Just do it" may just be your path to success. But for many of us, "Just do it" can feel too overwhelming. It can feel like you're about to dive into the deep end . . . with sharks.

While some people learn best by rolling up their shirtsleeves and diving right into the fray, I'm not one of them. Experience has taught me that if you want things to go smoothly in your hypnotherapy sessions, you need to set things up for them to happen.

Do you want clients you can be successful with?

Do you want to feel confident guiding a healing program?

Do you want to wrap up every session powerfully without ever needing a script?

If having to "just do it" feels like facing a firing squad for *you*, this book is for you. If you're the kind of person who needs more time to figure things out or to ease into the healing process more gently, I wrote this book for you. In it, I'm going to show you how to set up and wrap up your hypnotherapy sessions without ever needing a script.

You're about to discover simple, practical solutions that you can use right away to set yourself up to be more successful in facilitating a hypnotherapy program. These are things that helped me in my Regression Hypnotherapy practice. They helped me to feel more confident guiding the healing process, get paid a premium fee, and grow a referral-based business.

They can help you, too.

WHAT OTHERS SAY

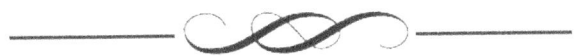

5 Out of 5 Stars!

"More wonderful words of wisdom from Wendie Webber in her second book, 'Ditch the Script.' Her expert teaching and guidance will benefit any hypnotherapist wishing to improve their regression skill and increase their confidence, no matter where they are on their journey. Wendie is an extremely knowledgeable, reputable and highly experienced Regression to Cause Hypnotherapist and hypnotherapy trainer who I hold in very high esteem. In addition, she has the ability to share her expertise in an enlightening and easy-to-follow way, in both of her books, which I highly recommend and give 5 out of 5 stars!
~ *Toni Mackenzie, Psychotherapist, Regression to Cause Hypnotherapist, Happiness Mentor, Mindset Coach, Bestselling Author of Your Flight to Happiness: A 7-Step Journey to Emotional Freedom, Transatlantic Media Correspondent for The Brooklyn Café TV, UK*

Filled with Valuable Information for the Practicing Hypnotist

"I have been in the field of Hypnosis technology for 37 years. I have conducted thousands of hypnotherapy sessions in my office as well as on national television shows. Wendie Webber's 'Ditch the Script' book is filled with valuable information for the practicing hypnotist and those of you who want to conduct successful regression therapy. 'Ditch the Script' really says it all. I can honestly say that I would recommend this book to any practicing therapist and anyone who is interested in regression therapy and non-script dependency."
~*Tom Silver, Tom Silver Institute of Hypnosis, author of How-to Book of Hypnotism, and Hypnotism – A Hypnosis Training & Techniques Manual – the Real Questions & Answers, tomsilver.com*

Travel Light with "A Mentor in Your Pocket"

"If you are a hypnotherapist, and you've read Wendie's first book 'The Devil's Therapy', or met Wendie on the internet or in person, you would have wished that you had a mentor like her when it comes to post-training challenges. Well, your wish has been granted. Wendie's new book 'Ditch the Script' is the answer. It is what I call 'a mentor in your pocket.' 'Ditch the Script' will save you time searching and worrying about the conventional stuff and makes sure it's not about the hypnosis, it's about the results. One thing is for sure . . . you will Ditch the Script after reading this book, you will travel light to your successful sessions, with only a blank piece of paper, a pen, and what you've gained from this book. Use it Wisely."
~Daniel Ghanime, MBA, DEHI Trainer, Counseling Hypnotherapist, Clinical Hypnoanalyst, Emotional Intelligence Development Specialist, Morphopsychologist, Parenting Coach, theControlAlt.com

Heart-Centered for the Client & Hypnotherapist

"This book offers a solid set-up to wrap-up to successfully navigate working with clients in a way that is not only heart-centered for the client but heart-centered for the hypnotherapist. She offers candidly, through her own experiences as a Healer, easy-to-follow steps to help you confidently and powerfully be the guide that your clients truly need. This book will help you transition from 'I'm not sure what I'm going to do with the client (panic!)' to 'I trust that I have the tools and knowledge, both internally and externally (easy breathing) to confidently guide my clients to successfully resolution of their issues.'"
~ Rosa Livingstone, CHt, Author of Self-Sabotage: The Art of Screwing Up, A Load Off Your Mind Coaching, Coquitlam, B.C.

You, too, Can Build a Successful Business

"As Wendie says, you need to feel confident in your ability to deliver on your promise of results. I appreciate how her books and courses are presented in steps. Learn from Wendie and deliver the best results possible for your clients, so you, too, can build a successful business."
~ Helena Jehnichen, Certified Clinical Hypnotherapist, The Stop Smoking Lady, Flourish Hypnosis, Canada

A Valuable Resource That Can Transform Your Practice

"This is 'that book' that stays on your work desk! My first experience with Wendie Webber was in a Facebook group where I answered a question with such technical brilliance and attention to terminological detail that it totally went over the head of the person reaching out for help. To see that person's response to Wendie's reply, by saying, 'I love how you know exactly how to explain complex things simply' taught me a valuable lesson . . . to keep it simple, stupid! Wendie has a way with words afforded only to those who have walked the walk to talk the talk. Being able to convert her extensive knowledge-based and superior intellect into words that resonate with the reader is a true gift. This book invites the reader to feel heard as she answers all the questions often not asked, but so needed, by new and seasoned practitioners, to bring about those client outcomes that all dedicated practitioners strive for." ~ *Scott Allerton, Sydney Integrative Hypnotherapy, Australia*

Helping the Practicing Hypnotist to Locate the Power of Hypnosis

"In her new book, 'Ditch the Script', Wendie Webber teaches you how to unlock your power as a hypnotist so you can help your clients find success. From my long career as a licensed clinical social worker, an attorney who has advocated exclusively on behalf of people with disabilities, a certified life coach, and a certified professional hypnotist, I understand the importance of finding, unlocking, and using your personal strength and gifts. In fact, my book, *Hurts So Good: An Orgasm of Tears*, fully explores how the human body sheds emotional tears to reach homeostasis, and how that physiological process beautifully parallels orgasm. In that same vein, Wendie Webber is an experienced practitioner who, in her new book, Ditch the Script, provides a similar lesson in helping the practicing hypnotist to locate the power of hypnosis, and how to access it. She distills down the potential snags you may have in helping clients to be successful, and teaches you how to face and disarm them. I recommend you buy Ditch the Script, read it, and use its lessons." ~ *Jayne M. Wesler, LCSW, Attorney, ICBCH-Certified NLP Practitioner and Life Coach, ICBCH-Certified Professional Hypnotist, and Author of Handbook for Parents of Children with Special Needs: A Therapeutic and Legal Approach; Hurts So Good: An Orgasm of Tears; Hurts So Good: An Orgasm of Tears Workbook; and No Bones About It: How to Increase Your Bone Density Without Medication*

Hippocrates taught that drugs should be used sparingly and only when absolutely necessary. Of course, in his day, there were only 268 known drugs, all herbal, and treatments were largely preventive medicine, but his first law of healing was – "Above all, don't make things worse." Today, this is known as the Hippocratic Oath.

~ *The Devil's Therapy*

CHAPTER 1:
Success is in Your Set Up

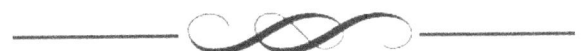

When you get a new client, how confident do you feel proceeding with them? You need to feel confident in your ability to deliver on your promise of results. That's what your clients are paying for. The secret to your success lies in your setup. It's in how well you set yourself up and your client to be successful working together. Setting yourself up for successful hypnotherapy sessions can give you the confidence you need to guide a healing process, even when you're not sure what to do. It can give you the time you need to take on even the most challenging issues or clients.

I've had clients who wouldn't follow instructions and clients who weren't *able* to relax. I've had clients who were so anxious that they couldn't keep their eyes closed for more than a few seconds at a time, and clients with so many problems that I felt completely out of my depth, just trying to figure out where to begin! I've had clients who would run away into past lives rather than face the truth of just how painful their childhood had been in *this* life. I've had clients who were so disconnected from their feelings that they couldn't, or wouldn't, let themselves feel anything. And then there have been clients who have had emotional meltdowns before they even sat down in the chair.

This is the kind of stuff that will drive you nuts if you don't know what to do. Then there's all the weird and creepy stuff. There are clients who see dead people, have experienced alien abductions, and those who can't sleep because there are things that go bump in the night. I've had more than one client turn into a "demon." I kid you not. Maybe it wasn't the Linda-Blair-pea-soup-spewing kind of thing but nasty, just the same.

I know what it's like to have stuff happen that you're not prepared for and how seriously it can throw you off your game. If you don't know where to begin or set up for the next step, you won't feel confident. That's a problem because if you don't feel confident in your sessions, your clients will sense it. A client in hypnosis is hyper-aware. If you're feeling nervous, they're going to pick up on it. If you have doubts, they're going to feel it, and they won't trust you enough to follow your instructions. You need them to follow instructions to get the results.

Your primary job is to make it safe for the client to follow your instructions. You can't do that if you don't feel confident. When you don't feel like you're in charge of your session, you'll start to lose your nerve. You'll begin to doubt yourself and your abilities. You might even begin to question whether or not you're even qualified to do this work. You'll be so worried about all the unknowns and everything that might go wrong or could go wrong that you won't be thinking about how you can help a person. You'll be focusing on all the what-ifs.

What if you take on more than you can handle? What if you get in over your head? What if you fuck up[1] and make a complete fool of yourself? When you start thinking this way, it's only a matter of time before you'll start to beat yourself up. You'll convince yourself that you don't know enough, that you're not good enough, that you need more tools or techniques when the truth is that *you feel afraid*. That's when you'll start to avoid. You'll start to procrastinate. You'll put things off. You'll find ways to distract yourself. And you'll avoid doing the regression work.

---

[1] If you don't like "bad" language, get over it. Your clients are going to use it and it's actually a good thing. "Bad" language has therapeutic value in your sessions so learn when to encourage it.

When fear blocks you, you won't get a lasting result. But what if I were to tell you there are just three things getting in your way? The three most common obstacles that get in the way of your ability to confidently guide a healing process and get results that last all have everything to do with how you *think*. Change how you think, and you'll get a different result. But you already knew that, right?

Obstacle #1 — The Hypnosis

Have you noticed how hypnosis forums seem to focus entirely on the hypnosis? When a practitioner posts a question, too often they have a new client coming in next week —or worse, tomorrow—and the hypnosis practitioner is in a panic because they have *no idea* what to do. Most of the time, they haven't even seen the client, and they're trying to figure out a treatment plan. The advice offered. A hypnotic technique, script, or process. Here's the problem: A professional healing practitioner is looking for a script or a protocol to help a person they have never met resolve a problem they know nothing about. Why? Because the practitioner thinks that hypnosis is the answer.

Change how you think about hypnosis.

People don't pay for hypnosis - they pay for results. While hypnosis is highly effective for a surprising number of painful problems, it's not the answer for every client or every problem. Hypnosis is not magic. It's a tool. In the hands of a skilled practitioner, it can be a powerful tool for creating real and lasting positive change. But there's no Power in hypnosis.

The *Power* is in the Mind of the client. You are uniquely qualified to help a person gain *access* to that Power. You can help them use that Power to dramatically change their lives for the better. But hypnosis is not the answer. *You are*. Most hypnosis training focuses on techniques and protocols because you need them. They are, after all, the tools of your trade. But the "secret sauce" isn't in the hypnosis. It's in your unique gifts and abilities. It's in your passion for helping people heal themselves, their relationships, and their lives. It's up to you to develop these things into skills to deliver them to your clients.

This begins with getting a firm handle on your existing tools and protocols. You don't need more tools. You need to master the ones you already have. What do they do? How do they work? When should you use this one rather than that one? Do you know? The more you master your methods, the more confident you'll feel in your sessions, and the better your results will be.

A common complaint I hear from many hypnosis practitioners is that basic certification taught them little to nothing about Regression Hypnotherapy. Some, myself included, were taught that regression is "bad." Let's set the record straight. Regression is neither good nor bad. It's simply a tool. Like any tool, its "goodness" lies in how skillfully you use it. Just as a scalpel can be used as an instrument of healing or a lethal weapon, and medicine can be used as a poison, it's all in how you use it. It's up to you to learn how to use it wisely.

I was fortunate to find Gerald Kein and Omni-Hypnosis early in my career. This gave me the foundation I needed to feel confident facilitating Regression Hypnotherapy. But I didn't stop there. I continued to invest in myself and in learning the tools of my trade. In the end, I learned from many of the top teachers in the hypnosis field, earning multiple certifications and receiving a couple of awards to boot. For example, Stephen Parkhill, author of *Answer Cancer*, taught me the importance of qualifying the client.

Alchemical Hypnotherapy, with David Quigley, showed me how Parts Work is a foundation for effective Regression Hypnotherapy. This understanding eventually led me to gain certification in Satir Transformational Systemic Therapy.

Cal Banyan's 5-PATH® and 7th Path Self-Hypnosis® taught me a more clinical approach to therapeutic hypnosis. Learning how to be more systematic in my approach was a game-changer in my sessions with clients.

Regression Hypnotherapy Boot Camp, with Matt Sison and Randy Shaw, showed me how emotional release work is the secret to real and lasting results. My experience at Boot Camp inspired me to write my first book, *The Devil's Therapy: Hypnosis Practitioner's Essential Guide to Effective Regression Hypnotherapy*.[2] This brought me full circle back to what had inspired me to study hypnosis in the first place—a book based on Hippocrates' *Healing Power of Nature*.

Hippocrates is considered the father of modern medicine. His most fundamental teaching was that the role of the healer is to release the blocks to healing. Hippocrates believed that the power to heal exists within each of us, that it's an intelligence that already knows how to heal, and that the job of a healer is to interfere with it as little as possible. He instructed his students to only use surgical and chemical interventions as a last resort. This is what we must do.

Hypnosis gives us access to the Part of the Mind that knows how to heal. You don't need to tell it what to do because it already knows what to do. What it needs is *space* to do it. This is the function and purpose of a healer. It's to provide the space needed for healing to happen.

Obstacle #2 — The Client

Most hypnosis practices are based on a single session model because that's how you learned things in basic training. You learned to facilitate one protocol or technique at a time. But clients want real results. If all you know how to do is a single session, you won't get the results. Worse, you'll be focused on how you can get more clients just so you can pay the bills. That's no way to make a living.

Change how you think about clients.

You don't need "more clients." You need clients you can be successful with that will help you to grow your confidence and skill. "More clients" just means having more problems to deal with. If you're just

---

[2] In my first book, I use a Grimm's Fairy Tale to illustrate a three-phase, seven-step protocol for effective regression to cause hypnosis. Through the story, you learn a systemic approach to Regression Hypnotherapy comprised of three distinct phases. Each phase lays the foundation for the next phase, giving you a very step-by-step approach to facilitating a healing program. The first phase is the Set-Up Phase. If you'd like a free infographic of the complete system, go to www.devilstherapy.com

starting out, you don't need more problems. You need experiences that will put some wins under your belt. This begins with qualifying your clients.

The first step to setting yourself up for success is in qualifying your clients. In chapters two and three, we'll look at how to put yourself in charge of the healing process by qualifying the client first.

Obstacle #3 — The Results

The goal of Regression Hypnotherapy is a complete cessation of unwanted symptoms and effortless permanence. But to go beyond symptom management can take more time. It requires a client-centered approach because healing isn't something you do. It's something that happens when the client is ready to let go of the problem.

Change how you think about results.

Your job isn't to fix anything. It's to recognize that the Subconscious Mind is doing exactly what it was designed to do. While symptoms bring a client into your office, they're not the real problem. Symptoms are merely the Subconscious Mind's way of alerting the Conscious Mind to the fact there *is* a problem. Through the healing process, you will guide the client to discover, for him or herself, what the *real* problem is. Then, together, you can find the most appropriate way to correct it.

The second step to setting yourself up for success is in establishing the Therapeutic Relationship. This is the purpose of your intake process. Your intake is not merely to establish rapport. It's to lay the foundation for an alliance that will empower you to achieve real and lasting results. In chapters four, five, and six, we'll look at how you can unpack the client's presenting issue, assess the client's readiness to proceed, and identify the vital information you need to guide the healing process confidently and effectively.

In Chapter 7, we'll look at the three key pieces of information you need in every Regression Hypnotherapy session and how you can use it to wrap up every session powerfully—without ever needing a script.

In Chapter 8, you'll learn how to set up for the Forgiveness Work while you're taking a history of the client's issue.

In Chapter 9, you'll learn how to wrap up each session powerfully without ever needing a script.

In Chapter 10, you'll learn how to set up for the client's next session before emerging the client from hypnosis. You'll also learn two preliminary check-in questions that help identify where the next step in the client's healing process needs to be.

Your Success is Always in Your Set Up

I want to change how you *think* in your hypnotherapy sessions. My earliest experience in life taught me to "look before you leap." Experience working with real clients who have real problems has taught me that it's not always prudent to dive into hypnosis right away. Just do it isn't always your best strategy.

The simple strategies you're about to learn will make your job easier by getting rid of problems you don't need. They can help you feel more confident in your Regression Hypnotherapy sessions by providing the information you need to guide the healing process effectively.

By the time you finish reading the last page, you'll know how to identify the right client for you, where to begin the healing process, what to pay attention to during the client's sessions, how to wrap up your sessions in a way that sets up for the next session, and where to begin the client's next session.

Ready to get started? Read on . . .

The client must be willing to allow feelings and emotions to be part of the process. Don't wipe away the truth of how you feel. Don't deny your deepest feelings. Tears — whether of sadness, anger, grief, or joy — must be brought to conscious awareness and allowed to express. ~ **The Devil's Therapy**

CHAPTER 2:
Qualify Your Clients

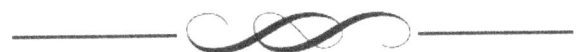

When you're just starting out, it's a temptation to try to sell the session right away. But when a person calls and asks, "How much?" or "How many sessions?" they're asking the wrong question. They don't know anything about you or what you do. They just think all hypnosis is alike. They don't know that hypnosis is not the answer—*you* are.

You can't be all things to all people. Not everyone who calls you is going to be a client you can be successful with. To deliver on your promise of results, you need to assess whether or not they're the right client for you. You need to qualify your clients because no two clients are ever alike. They can come to you with the same symptom, but it's never the same problem. No two smokers are alike. No two weight problems are alike. No two anxiety clients are alike. This is because every problem is the result of a life experience. It has everything to do with the client's history.

Some clients will come to you with a surface issue. Surface issues respond well to surface techniques like suggestion and guided imagery. For example, stress eating or blocks to academic, sports, or vocational performance can often be resolved in one to three sessions with suggestions alone. The problem is that hypnosis is seldom the first solution people turn to when they have a problem. It's not until the problem has been around for a while, decades often, that they decide to "try" hypnosis. By then, the problem has had time to grow and evolve, and it's not a simple issue anymore. It's a painful, persistent problem which means you've got your work cut out for you.

What's the problem?

Anxiety disorders, panic attacks, irrational fears, angry outbursts, prolonged grief, addictive behaviors, and chronic physical conditions are deeper issues. They have to do with unresolved memories from the past that continue to generate physical and emotional pain. You can't merely suggest away an emotion. Why would you even try? Emotions are not the problem. Emotions are just one of the ways the Subconscious Mind communicates with the Conscious Mind.

Symptoms are how the Subconscious Mind communicates with the Conscious Mind. The lump, bump, ache, pain, knee-jerk reactivity, pervasive mood, irrational emotions and responses, driven behavior, etc., are how Subconscious Mind brings attention to an underlying problem that's calling for resolution. When surface approaches fail to get a lasting result, it's usually because you're dealing with a deeper issue.

Symptoms are what motivate a person to seek out your help, but they're seldom the whole problem. When the client's issue is emotional, it won't respond to surface approaches because the symptom isn't the problem. It's a Subconscious solution to the *real problem*, which has to do with an unresolved past experience. This is why you must never try to get rid of the symptom. Any attempt to eliminate, override, suppress or remove the symptom without resolving the underlying problem will, at best, result in temporary relief. If you try to use a surface technique on a deeper issue, you might be able to manage the symptoms, but it won't resolve the problem. In some cases, it can even make the problem worse by reinforcing the Conscious Mind's avoidance strategy.

Avoiding doesn't make the problem go away. Antidepressants don't get rid of depression. Relaxation techniques don't get rid of the anxiety. Ego strengthening suggestions don't get rid of self-deprecating beliefs. Reminding the client of the cost of substance abuse won't stop the behavior. Imagining yourself standing up to a bully won't instill courage. You have to deal with the feeling. Unwanted feelings and emotions don't come out of nowhere. They come out of specific life experiences.

Healing happens given the right conditions. Your job is to create those conditions. It begins by assessing whether a person is the right client for you. You need to assess:

1. The problem
2. The client
3. Yourself

Regression Hypnotherapy is not for everyone. It's not for every issue. And not every client is going to be right for you. You need to feel confident guiding a client through a healing program. For this reason, you cannot afford to work with just anyone. If you try to take on more than you're ready for, you'll soon find yourself in over your head. When that happens, you won't know what to do. You'll start to feel afraid. When you get stuck, you'll struggle to get results. You can avoid problems that you just don't need simply by qualifying your clients.

Here's how to think about it. Every person who calls to inquire about your services is applying for the position of being your client. Hypnotherapy requires a relationship. That's what you're qualifying your clients for—a Therapeutic Relationship. The Therapeutic Relationship doesn't begin with the client's first session with you. It begins with your first conversation.

To qualify your clients, you need to have a conversation. The purpose of the initial conversation is not to take a comprehensive history of the client's issue. It's simply to help the person to feel more comfortable talking with you and to qualify whether or not this is the right client for you.

When a caller asks, "How much?" or "How many sessions?" you can initiate a conversation by saying, "I'll be happy to answer all your questions. Would it be alright if I ask *you* a few questions first?" The client's permission marks the beginning of the Therapeutic Relationship.

The 3 Rs in R-R-Results

The 3 Rs in R-R-Results is a simple preliminary testing technique you can use to quickly assess if a person is the right client for you. If they are, you can continue into a more in-depth conversation about the problem and how you can help.

Reasonable

The first R is "**R**easonable." Is it reasonable to expect that the presenting issue can be resolved with hypnosis?

Hypnosis is not a cure-all. You need to establish realistic expectations regarding what's possible. For example, I once had a client ask me to erase all her bad memories. They have drugs that can do that now, but even if I *could* do it, I wouldn't because our past experiences have value. The goal of Regression Hypnotherapy is to put an end to the pain of the past by putting an end to avoidance strategies. Erasing or burying the past doesn't get rid of it. It just drives it deeper into the Subconscious Mind, where it will continue to wreak havoc in the client's daily life. It's through facing the past that painful experiences can be transformed into a source of empowerment and healing for the client.

Is the client expecting a single-session fix? If so, they're likely to be disappointed. Yes, one-session miracles can and do happen but, if you're just starting, it's an unrealistic expectation. It takes confidence, skill, experience, and a measure of luck to deliver a lasting result in a single session. You need to be realistic. If you're starting in your practice, you lack experience, and you're still developing your knowledge and skill. Having to deliver miracles on demand puts too much pressure on you. You don't need that!

When it comes to helping real clients with real issues, a single session is seldom enough to get the job done. If the problem has been around for a while, it's reasonable to expect that it might take a while to back the client out of it. The symptoms are merely what the Conscious Mind is aware of. They're not the whole problem. The underlying problem is at the Subconscious level of the Mind. That's where you need to go to resolve the problem. But you won't know what the real problem is or how long it will take to resolve it until you get the client into hypnosis and ask their Subconscious Mind to show you.

Healing can take time because the Power isn't in the hypnosis or the technique. It's in the Mind of the client. Being client-centered means recognizing that the time it takes isn't up to you. It's up to the client. There can be resistance coming from the Conscious Mind. There can be Subconscious resistance. It's not just reasonable to give the client whatever time she needs to allow healing to happen, and it's a kindness.

The first R in R-R-Results is "**R**easonable." When a person comes to you with an issue, the first assessment is, "What are this person's expectations regarding the process? Are they reasonable?"

Right

The second R in Results is "**R**ight." "Is this the right client *for you?*" Is it reasonable to expect that you can be successful working with this person? It's simply not reasonable to expect to be all things to all people.

For the Therapeutic Relationship to work, there needs to be a *match* between you and the client. While hypnotherapy has been proven to be highly effective with a multitude of mental, emotional and behavioral symptoms, not every client is necessarily the right client for you. You need to stay within the scope of your training and experience. The client's issue should be a fit for your qualifications. For example, a person who is experiencing acute pain, psychotic episodes, or suicidal thoughts needs to seek proper medical attention *first*.

Problems with addiction are complex issues. They're not suited to new practitioners. Serious mental disorders are no place for you to get your feet wet. It's not that hypnosis can't help these people, but you need to know your limits. If the client's problem is beyond the scope of your knowledge and experience, refer them out. Realize they're just not the right client for you *at this time*.

Hypnosis is awesome for things like pain management and smoking cessation. But what if they're calling about a bi-polar condition? Or schizophrenia? Or obsessive-compulsive disorder (OCD)? Or general anxiety disorder (GAD)? What about self-mutilation behavior? Or cancer? Or irritable bowel syndrome (IBS)? While many of these issues can be resolved with therapeutic hypnosis, the question is, is it reasonable to expect that *you* can resolve these things using hypnosis?

If you're fresh out of the classroom, you are probably not ready to deal with the more complex and challenging issues mentioned above. That's because complex issues can be . . . complex. Complex issues have a lot of moving parts. For example, fibromyalgia is a syndrome. It's a collection of symptoms that are all clustered together. That means complexity. If you don't know what to do, it can be confusing. Confusion kills confidence.

Confidence is a lot like a muscle. It gets stronger with practice. But if you try to take on more than you can handle before you're ready, you'll injure yourself. I used to manage a gym, so I know a little something about weightlifting. Just like at the gym, it's always best to start with lighter-weight issues. Over time you'll build up your strength. Before long, you'll be able to take on more challenging problems.

People are complex. Even when it's a simple problem, there can be hidden issues. What if your smoking cessation prospect also happens to suffer from schizophrenia or is bipolar or has depression? That's fine if it's an unrelated condition. But what if the smoking problem is connected to another condition? Are you the right choice for that person? What if the person just plain creeps you out? Do you even like the person? Do you want to work with them? This is important because rapport is critical to the healing process.

Ditch the Script

Rapport has to go both ways. If a prospective client sets off your "spidey senses," creeps you out, or has strong beliefs or biases that conflict with your own deeply held values or beliefs, you need to honor that. It's very difficult to treat a client with unconditional regard when you don't feel comfortable with them. For example, I had a guy call with a problem of obsessive-compulsive masturbation. While he was talking to me on the phone, he was "whacking off." To be honest, I wasn't comfortable with that. I was still fairly new. I wasn't prepared for it, and the guy creeped me out.

My heart goes out to him now. I recognize that he was in pain. He was just trying to find some help. But, at that time, I wasn't the right person to help him. I recognized that I didn't have enough experience to feel confident working with this issue, and I referred him out. Today, my response might be different, but this client and this issue were *not* a match for my knowledge and skill at that time. We weren't "right" for each other.

The BC Liquor Board has a saying, "Know your limit, stay within it." When it comes to healing work, it's important to know your limit. Know what you're qualified to take on. And trust your gut. It's not reasonable to expect that you can be all things to all people. We're all at different stages of evolution. To be successful in working with more challenging issues requires experience. In time, you'll get there. Give yourself permission to gain the experience you need to feel strong enough to take on the more challenging issues. When you have a solid foundation of knowledge and skill, you'll find that the scope of your practice expands considerably. The more you know your stuff, the more issues there are that become "reasonable" for you to take on.

The second R in R-R-Results is "**R**ight." Is this the right client for you? Are they a match for your present knowledge, skill, experience, beliefs? Do *you* even like them? Do you *want* to work with them?

Ready

The third R in Results is "**R**eady." Is the client ready, willing, and able to do the work necessary to achieve the results they are after? This is important because *you can't do it for them*. After all, it's their Mind! Is the client willing to go where you need them to go to get the results? Or do they expect you to do all the work while they lay back and relax? What if their doctor or spouse told them they have to quit smoking? What if they're just calling you to get somebody off their back?

It doesn't matter how ready *you* might be. What matters is whether the client is ready. If the client isn't ready to make the change, you can't make them. No one can. Hypnosis is not magic. A person has to be highly motivated to get the results they're after. To access the power to heal, the person needs to be ready to participate in their own healing.

The third R in R-R-Results is "**R**eady." Is the client ready to be an active participant in their own healing process? Are they prepared to do the work necessary to be successful working with you?

Summary

Qualifying your clients can help you to get the best possible outcomes for your hypnosis clients by giving you the foundation you need for successful hypnotherapy. It begins with the 3 Rs in R-R-Results. The 3 Rs allow you to quickly assess whether you want to continue the conversation with a prospective new client.

1. Reasonable?
2. Right?
3. Ready?

If the client's presenting issue is something that can *reasonably* be addressed with hypnosis, you're confident that you are the *right* healing practitioner to work with the client's issue, and the client isn't expecting you to wave your magic wand and erase all their bad memories, the next step is to invite your caller to talk more about the presenting problem.

CHAPTER 3:
Critical Qualifying Questions

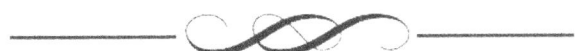

In my first book, *The Devil's Therapy: Hypnosis Practitioner's Essential Guide to Effective Regression Hypnotherapy*, I introduced a modern approach to facilitating therapeutic hypnosis. This is not a technique-focused or therapist-focused approach. It's a client-centered approach that keeps the focus on the body. This is because regression hypnotherapy works with emotional issues, and emotions are experienced physically.

Regression Hypnotherapy focuses on unresolved emotions trapped in past experiences, which are responsible for generating unwanted symptoms. Often, these unresolved events involve trauma. Trauma expert Dr. Robert Scaer has defined trauma as the perception of threat while in a state of helplessness. Helplessness is the natural state of the child. As a result, most of the issues we work with will have their roots in childhood.

Trauma is an unavoidable fact of life growing up. It's nature's way of developing resilience, but a traumatic experience remains unresolved; it disconnects a person from themselves and their truest emotions. Healing requires a change in consciousness. All healing is self-healing. It's not something you do. It's something that happens, given the right conditions. To facilitate a self-healing process requires attunement to the needs of the client because Regression Hypnotherapy is an experiential process that requires the client's participation. It is a permission-based approach where your job is to make it safe for the client to allow change to happen.

You can't make a person heal. Change occurs when the client makes a conscious decision based on understanding *now*. Without understanding, there can be no lasting result. Your job is to act as a guide, provide safety, and shine a light on the way through. It's never to diagnose, prescribe, or try to fix. It is to support and empower the client in discovering the answers to questions and solutions to problems that, consciously, have eluded him or her. You can then validate change when it happens.

To facilitate change, real change requires an attitude of compassion, not sympathy. You must guide, not lead, and let the answers be revealed through the process. This begins with a preliminary assessment process. Because Regression Hypnotherapy is a permission-based approach, it begins with asking permission to have a conversation. Most people will feel relieved that you've taken charge of the conversation because they don't really know what to ask. They don't know you. They really don't know what you do. As a result, they don't feel comfortable talking about themselves. They need to feel comfortable with you before they'll be willing to reveal their deepest, darkest secrets.

You're not drilling them for answers. This isn't an intake. Don't turn it into one. You're just having a conversation to assess whether or not you want to work together. What this conversation should tell you is how best to respond to this individual. It gives you the information you need to make what you do relevant to the person's issue. It's also an effective sales technique. The more you can get a person engaged in conversation with you, the more comfortable they will feel sharing things about themselves, and the more likely they will be to book the session. That's the goal, right?

Preliminary Assessment Questions

The following preliminary assessment questions can help your prospective client feel more comfortable talking about themselves and their problem.

The first three questions allow you to quickly assess whether or not you need to *continue* the conversation with them.

1. What's the problem?
2. Why is it a problem?
3. How much of a problem is it?

Many people are struggling simply because they don't feel heard. They're frustrated or despondent because no one has taken the time to listen. Show that you're different by listening. Demonstrate that you care by validating where they're at and how they feel. Let the client speak! This makes it safe for them to talk more intimately about the problem. Often, the experience of simply being heard can result in a much deeper realization of how they're truly feeling (and how much they want to get the problem resolved.) The more they talk about themselves, the more they will feel that they know you, and the more invested they will become in working with you. This is the first stage in establishing rapport.

1. What's the problem?

As far as the client is concerned, this is the most important question because this is the reason for seeking your help. The client always thinks that the symptoms are the problem. They just want to get rid of the ache, pain, lump, bump, unwanted behavior, or emotion. It's important that you honor this need and, whenever possible, offer hope. But remember that what the client thinks is the problem is just the perceived problem. It's seldom the real problem.

Symptoms form the basis of the client's Therapeutic Goal. They can provide you with a way to test your results. But they're not the whole problem. If they were, the client wouldn't be struggling to resolve it. Symptoms are merely the Conscious Mind's point of view. That's what's causing the client pain, so that's where you need to keep the focus—on the pain of the problem. Feelings are the territory of our Subconscious Mind. That's where you work!

The Subconscious Mind is the largest part of our consciousness, and yet, too many people don't know that it's normal to feel uncomfortable feelings. They were taught early in life to suck it up and be "tough little soldiers." As a result, the tendency is to try to minimize the discomfort. This just makes things worse because there's nowhere for the feelings to go.

With nowhere to go, the feelings trapped inside tend to build up over time, making the Subconscious Mind a pressure cooker. Eventually, the internal pressure gets to be too great, and that's when symptoms erupt into consciousness.

2. Why is this a problem?

Keep the caller focused on *why* they're calling. What's the problem they're struggling with? Why is it a problem? What's the pain they are in that they need relief from? If it's not something that can reasonably be resolved with hypnosis or something you're not qualified to work with, or if it's not something you want to work with, then there's no need to discuss things further. Refer them out. If it *is* something you can help them with, the next step is to get them to share more about themselves and the problem. Ask, "How long have you been struggling with this problem?"

If the client says that the problem is connected to a specific event, like a car accident or the death of a loved one, you have just opened the door to having a conversation about how feelings are connected to past events.

If they tell you that they've had this problem their whole life, you have just opened the door to talking about how problems are often rooted in childhood.

3. How much of a problem is this?

To be successful, you need clients who are highly motivated. The greater the pain, the greater the motivation to get the problem resolved. What happened to motivate them to call now?

Maybe they just reached the end of their rope. Maybe they have a special event coming up, like a wedding, and they want to look good for it. Maybe they want to quit smoking before the baby arrives. Maybe they've just gotten a diagnosis. On the other hand, maybe they're dealing with a chronic condition, have tried everything else, and they're desperate. How is having this problem impacting them in daily life? For example, how is the weight problem impacting them? How is the health problem impacting them? How is being afraid of X impacting other areas of their life?

This question can help the client to realize just how much of a problem it is for them because there's the problem, and then there are all the side-effects of having the problem. Having to *deal* with the problem on a daily basis just adds to the problem. These things tend to stack up over time. The longer they stack up, the more internal pressure there is looking for a way out. Remember, pain is the motivating factor. Human beings are hardwired to avoid pain. The more pain there is, the greater the motivation to resolve the problem. Helping the client to identify just how uncomfortable they are feeling can help them realize how important it is to get some relief.

If it doesn't sound like it's that much of a problem for the client, take a SUD. SUD stands for **S**ubjective **U**nit of **D**iscomfort (SUD). For example, "On a scale of one to ten, where ten is "the worst" it's ever been, how bad is it?"

Get the client to tell you because if they're only calling to appease their wife, or because Mom made them, or the doctor said they should, it's not really their idea. If it's not their idea, they're probably not all that motivated. You need your clients to be highly motivated, so ask. "On a scale of one to ten, how much of a problem is this?" Or, "On a scale of one to ten, how uncomfortable is this for you?" Or, "On a scale of one to ten, where ten is totally unbearable, how bad is it?" If their SUD is a seven or less, you might want to see if you can bring the intensity up before you go any further. For example, if the client's SUD level is a five, that's just not high enough for you to expect to be successful with them. In this case, you could ask, "What would need to happen for you to get it up to a ten?" You could engage the client's imagination. "What does life look like in three months' time, or six months or a year down the road, and nothing had changed?"

If these methods fail to increase their motivation, and their SUD is still less than a seven, it's possible they're expecting you to fix them. You can't. Hypnosis is not magic. It can seem that way, sometimes, but the magic is in the Mind of the client, not the hypnosis. If your prospective client can't get the intensity level above a seven, they're not ready yet. They're not sufficiently motivated to qualify as your client. The power to create a real and lasting change resides in the client's own Subconscious Mind. You can help them to access that power, but you can't *make* them change.

It wasn't until I was in my fifth year of practice that I finally got this. Your investment in the outcome should never be greater than the clients. If it is, you're sunk. The client is responsible for the results. You can guide the process. You can make it safe for the client to go where you need them to go to find the healing. But you can't do it for them.

Don't agree to work with just anyone. Don't waste your time on dabblers or people who want to "try" hypnosis or who expect you to do all the work. Make sure that your clients are every bit as committed as you are before agreeing to take them on as a client.

The higher the number, the higher the motivation. If the client says, "Oh, it's a TWELVE!" that's a highly motivated client. That's a client you can be successful with!

4. What can you tell me about hypnosis?

Once you have qualified that the client is motivated, invite the client to tell you what they know about hypnosis. What do they think hypnosis is? How do they think it can help them? What are their expectations with respect to hypnosis? Are they realistic? Are they reasonable? Most people have misconceptions about what happens in a hypnosis session. This gives you the opportunity to uncover any erroneous ideas they might have and correct them before the client shows up for their first session. If you uncover some specific worries or concerns, talk about how your approach is different from what they expected. This, then, opens the door to talking about how you work and what your fee is.

During your preliminary assessment conversation, your client has been revealing their innermost self with you. You've made it safe for them to be vulnerable with you and share their Pain Story. This is the perfect time to book the session but before you discuss your fee, say, "You probably have some questions for me . . ." And wait.

5. You probably have some questions for me . . .

Allow a moment of silence for the client to respond because they might just disclose something that could be critical to their healing. Then, do a quick review to verify that you understand the client's intended goal. For example, "So, as I understand it … (this is the problem) … (this is your goal)."

Remind them of the painful feelings associated with the problem. Then, shift the energy to establish positive expectancy toward working with you. Ask how resolving *that* problem might help them in daily life. Let the *client* sell you on the benefits of change.

This is the time to educate your client about what to expect when they show up for their first session with you. Get them to imagine what it will be like to be there with you. For example, my first session is what I call a "Set for Success" session. The purpose of this first session is assessment. This allows me to design a program that is suited to the client's specific needs. What's going to happen? Three things.

First, I take a complete history of the client's problem. Second, I teach them what they need to know to be successful working with me. Third, I guide them through a short hypnosis session. This is, of course, an extreme simplification, but it's a proven system that gets rid of a load of resistance before you start regressing a client into painful past events.

Having a first session to kick off a healing program puts you in the driver's seat of the process. It also gets rid of the unrealistic expectation of a single-session fix.

You can learn more in the Ready for Regression First Session System Course. https://www.tribeofhealers.com/ready-for-regression-first-session-system-course/

Regression Hypnotherapy isn't a single session approach. Your preliminary conversation should make this clear. Even if you resolve the client's issue in the first session, you won't know if it's completely resolved unless you test your results in the client's daily life. For example, I once met a guy in a social situation. When he learned that I was a hypnosis practitioner, he was excited to tell me all about how much he loves hypnosis. He then proceeded to tell me about his celebrity hypnotherapist, who has her own radio show. She clearly had a prestige which he was borrowing through his association with her. Apparently, she had helped him twenty years ago to quit smoking. He just couldn't say enough about how great she was.

Then he lit up a cigarette. Wait. What?

His hypnotherapist probably boasts a 99% success rate. The question is, for how long? The truth is, to get a lasting result, you must test. It can take time to clean out all the aspects contributing to the client's problem. People are not machines. You can't just take them apart and put them back together again and expect them to run perfectly. Human beings are complex organisms. No two are alike. Each needs to be treated with care because change doesn't come easily for most of us. It takes time to accept and then integrate change fully. Testing is how you get a lasting result. Even if you deliver a one-session miracle, you need at least one follow-up session to verify that the issue is completely resolved. Set this up ahead of time.

Once you have addressed the client's expectations and concerns about the process, verified their intended goal and benefits, it's time to schedule your client for their first session. Unfortunately, this is where a lot of healing practitioners get stuck. They don't feel comfortable discussing their fee, and they find it difficult to ask for a commitment to the first session. They're afraid of sounding "salesy." This is where Qualifying Question #6 gets you off the hook.

6. If you were to proceed with me, ideally, how soon would you like to get started?

That's it. Simple, right? This is a no-sweat, no-pressure way to book the session because it takes selling right out of the equation. Qualifying Question #6 makes booking the first session easy because the client isn't faced with too many choices. The only choice they have to make is, how soon do they want to get started?

Don't complicate things. Just get a commitment to the first session. If they're ready to proceed, you can sort out how they wish to pay. Then, schedule them in for their first session. And that's all you ever need to sell a person—the first session. Your first session gives you and the client the opportunity to decide whether or not you want to *continue* to work together. If for any reason, you don't feel that this is going to be the best approach for them, you have an out. In either case, most people notice a positive shift, even after the first session. That's what will sell them on the process, so you won't have to. But the objective is to set the client up to enjoy lasting results, not just short-term success.

The first step in the healing journey is to commit to the first step. You won't know what you're dealing with until you guide the client through the first session. If following the first session, you and the client decide to continue working together, that's the time to offer a multi-session package. Until then, there's no need to offer more than the first session. This takes the pressure off both you and the client because it's just one small commitment. This is the secret to your success. All you ever need to focus on is setting up for the next step. When the client successfully takes that step, you focus on the next step.

Summary

Qualifying your clients isn't about selling or "making the sale." It's about interviewing a person to see if you're a good fit. If you think of a caller as someone who is applying for the position of a client, you won't feel like you're trying to sell them anything. As a result, you'll feel much more relaxed and confident while having the initial conversation with a prospective new.

Once you have established the 3 Rs in R-R-Results, that the issue is something that can reasonably be resolved with hypnotherapy, that the client is right for you, a match for your level of knowledge and skill, and that the client is sufficiently motivated to be ready to participate in a healing process, all you need is a commitment to the first session.

Your preliminary conversation should clarify that Regression hypnosis isn't a single session approach. It's a client-centered approach based on the client's needs. Healing requires a relationship. That's what you're qualifying your clients for—the Therapeutic Relationship.

With some people, you'll know right away, especially when they're *not* a good fit. That's when you can avoid problems you don't need by referring them out. With others, you might feel confident that you can help them, but you won't know, for sure, until you facilitate the first session.

The first session gives you the opportunity to conduct a thorough intake, guide the client into hypnosis, and take a look "under the hood." Until you do that, you won't know what you're dealing with. Not really. The six qualifying questions give you a way to assess whether a person is the right client for you, whether you're the right healer for them, and whether you're ready to begin a healing journey together.

CHAPTER 4:
Take a History

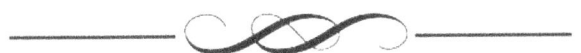

The intake is a pre-hypnosis interview where your focus is on taking a client history. This marks the beginning of the healing journey you and the client will take together and, used strategically, can help you to uncover the vital information you need to guide the healing process.

The first step in the healing process is always to find the feeling. "That feeling," whether it be fear, sadness, anger, or something else, is directly connected to the event that caused it to form in the first place. It's a signal transmitting from the initial sensitizing event (ISE). The client may be experiencing this signal as a feeling of tension or tightness in the body. It may be a physical ache or an emotional pain. It might be an unwanted behavior. Whatever it is, "the problem" has roots in the client's history.

I was taught not to waste any time talking with the Conscious Mind. The reasoning was that if the Conscious Mind doesn't know how to resolve the problem, why waste time listening to it? The Subconscious Mind has the information needed to resolve the client's issue, so that's where we need to go. Conclusion? Just get the client into hypnosis quickly and go to work. In other words, "Just do it."

Here's the problem . . . Hypnosis merely gives you access to the Subconscious level of Mind. *Healing* requires the client's participation. You need the client to be willing to go where you need them to go and do what you need them to do when you instruct them to do so. That takes trust. The problem is that rapport isn't a given. It must be earned. If you try to guide a person into hypnosis before they're ready, you're going to have to deal with unnecessary resistance.

Authoritarian approaches may be suitable for entertainment purposes, such as stage hypnotism or street hypnosis, but healing requires a relationship of trust. When you're dealing with an emotional issue, you need to take the time to listen to what the Conscious Mind has to say. Listening is a strategy. It's a way for you to set yourself up for success because it's not just about listening. It's about getting a person's Subconscious Mind to work *with* you. That's the basis of the Therapeutic Relationship.

The Therapeutic Relationship

People who have struggled with an issue a long time sometimes aren't just dealing with the problem. They're packing a load of frustration and anger, and depression on top of the problem. This is especially true of clients who have been through the medical mill. The healthcare system is focused on diagnosing and treating the symptoms—not the client. The patient's state of mind is largely ignored, even though that's the key to healing. You can relieve a ton of that pressure simply by satisfying the Conscious Mind's need to be heard. Not only can this give you a client who is easier to work with, but it can also help you to get better results.

Hypnosis is seldom the first solution most people turn to when they have a painful, persistent problem. If the client has been let down by other therapies, they're not going to find it easy to trust you or the process. To undo this negative bias, you need to earn the client's trust before you get them into hypnosis. If you don't, the client will just carry it into the hypnosis session with them.

Some clients will not be as forthcoming as you need them to be. Exposing shameful truths makes them feel uncomfortable. If they grew up in an environment of criticism and abuse, they won't feel safe opening up to a complete stranger. As a result, they'll withhold information that might be critical to their healing. They may even project irrational fears based on abusive past relationships onto you. The Therapeutic Relationship should be a safe place for the client to expose the dark underbelly of their Subconscious Mind.

Therapeutic hypnosis requires an alliance between therapist and client because you need the client's cooperation to get to the underlying cause of the problem. Every client needs to know that they can trust you with their deepest, darkest secrets, that what they share with you is in strictest confidence. They need to know that nothing they say would ever shock you and that you would never judge or bully them. They need you to be a trusted ally. Only then will they feel safe enough to let you guide them into uncharted territory.

Set Up for the Therapeutic Contract

The Subconscious Mind's primary concern is the client's survival. Its job is to protect the client. Your job is to work *with* the Subconscious Mind. You do this by making it safe for the client to follow your instructions. This is the purpose of the Therapeutic Contract.

The Therapeutic Contract gives you permission to do your job by establishing an agreement, between you and the client, regarding who does what. Think of it as the Rules of Conduct for therapy. Your side of the agreement is to care, protect and guide the client safely through a healing process. The client agrees to *let* you guide them by following your instructions. While this agreement is secured during the educational pre-talk, the process of establishing the Therapeutic Contract begins during the intake.

The Therapeutic Relationship lays the foundation for the Therapeutic Contract. This is why the intake process comes first. The intake allows you to customize your educational pre-talk to the specific needs and concerns of each individual client. Some hypnotherapists rely on canned pre-talks and online intake forms because these strategies save the therapist time. But taking the time to listen to the client's Pain Story can save time when you most need it by establishing rapport with *both* the Conscious and Subconscious minds. This is a more client-centered approach to preparing a client for hypnotherapy.

Make It Safe

The Conscious Mind and Subconscious Mind both want the same thing—safety. It's just that they have different strategies for accomplishing this. As both are integral to the client's well-being, you need to work with both. Your intake process can be a way to make it safe for both the Conscious and Subconscious minds to cooperate in the healing process.

The Subconscious Mind naturally communicates with the Conscious Mind through images, pictures, memories, emotions, and sensations in the body. When the Conscious Mind tries to suppress, repress or avoid in an attempt to control the Subconscious Mind, it puts these two parts of the client at odds with one another. There's a conflict. Your job is to get these two parts of the client working together by improving communication between them. To bring these two parts of the client back into alignment, you cannot dismiss one side in favor of the other. One is not better than the other. You need to listen to both.

Freud's Iceberg Mind Model depicts the Conscious Mind as the tip of the iceberg while the Subconscious Mind is the far-greater part of the Mind beneath the surface. But just as the brain has two hemispheres, which constantly communicate with one another, the Conscious Mind and Subconscious Mind are not separate entities. Each performs different functions and communicates very differently, but there is no real separation between these two parts of the client. It's one Mind.

The Conscious Mind is the part of the client that relies on thinking, reasoning, and logic to make sense of the world. This provides the client with a much-needed sense of control. If you don't satisfy the client's need to understand before you begin the induction process, the Conscious Mind will just try to run the show. When that happens, the client will be preoccupied with thinking, analyzing, and trying to figure things out. Unfortunately, this will only get in your way and block you from making progress.

To the Conscious Mind, control equals safety. The problem is that, consciously, the client doesn't have control in some area of their life. That's why they need you. It's the Subconscious Mind that has the control. The Pain Story only tells you the Conscious Mind's Story, what the Conscious Mind *thinks* about the problem. The rest of the Story belongs to the Subconscious Mind. To gain access to that information, you need to gain the trust of the Subconscious Mind. The Subconscious Mind is the emotional part of the Mind. It doesn't think, it feels, and it is duty-bound to protect the client from any perceived threat. If you don't earn its trust, the Subconscious Mind will try to protect the client *from you*. It will block you.

While you are talking with the Conscious Mind, the Subconscious Mind isn't off somewhere. It's right there with you, doing what it does best - assessing the situation for safety. It's watching you carefully to determine whether or not you can be trusted based on how you interact with the client. If you want the Subconscious Mind to cooperate with you, you need to show it that you're someone who will listen to how the client *feels*.

Your attitude needs to be easy-going and non-judgmental. Make it more of a conversation than an interview. It's not an interrogation. It's about getting to know the client a little better and showing that you care. Prove that you're not a threat. You're here to help. This allows the Subconscious Mind to feel safe and relax. When the Subconscious relaxes, it's like the family dog who just loves you. You can break into the house, and it will show you where all the bones are buried.

Hypnosis Happens

Taking a history of the client's problem is naturally going to stir up thoughts and feelings. As the client is telling you their Pain Story, they'll be remembering people and situations from the past and connecting with feelings and emotions that are related to their issue. What part of the Story holds the feeling? What emotion are they experiencing as they talk about those things? Who are they blaming? This is valuable information that can help you to guide the process. The more you help a client to connect with the pain of their Story, the more they'll start feeling emotions. When this happens, you have Critical Faculty By-Pass. That's hypnosis! The more intensity of feeling there is, the deeper the client is going into the Subconscious Mind. This can give you deep hypnosis.

Pay attention because, most of the time, the client will already be in hypnosis by the time you begin the induction. You just need to formalize it. That's what the induction procedure is. It's a ritual. A formal induction satisfies the client's need to know that they were hypnotized. That's what the client thinks they're paying you for. But the hypnosis will often happen long before you start the induction process. All you have to do is watch for it. The moment you notice a sign of emotion coming to the surface, bring attention to it. Show that you won't judge, that you're not a threat by validating that feeling. Encourage it. Give the feeling permission to be there. This will deepen the hypnosis by increasing rapport with the Subconscious Mind. For example, "There's the feeling! That feeling is allowed to be there! Realize that has everything to do with the reason you're here. You're allowed to feel it!"

When you validate a feeling, you are speaking directly to the Subconscious Mind. That's where the pain is coming from. It's coming out of the event that caused it. Emotions that arise during the intake process are not coming from what's happening in your office. They are bubbling up from the Subconscious level of Mind, where all the client's memories and emotions are stored.

When an emotional memory comes to Mind, that experience is connected to the client's presenting issue. The Subconscious Mind knows how the problem got started. When a feeling comes to the surface, that's the Subconscious Mind speaking. Giving the feeling permission to be there is a way of validating the Subconscious Mind. You are showing it that, unlike the rest of the world, you value what it has to say. You're not here to shut it down. You're here to listen because you understand that the Subconscious Mind isn't the enemy. It wants what's best for the client. *And so do you.* You're here to help the client get what they need. This is how you form an alliance with the client's Subconscious Mind.

Form an Alliance

Some clients have pretty gritty stories to share. They'll have conscious memories of trauma and abuse. They'll have painful grievances with loved ones who hurt them. Sharing these experiences with a complete stranger can make the client feel vulnerable. It can bring up shame. Shame is not a feeling. It's a thought. It's a belief that says, "I'm flawed and irreparably broken. There's something wrong with me. I'm worthless, don't deserve. I'm unlovable."

No matter what the client shares with you, demonstrate that nothing they could say would ever shock you. You've heard it before, it's sad but true, and you won't be the one to judge them. Make it safe for the client to face the truth of how they feel. If the client becomes highly emotional, that's okay. That's their Subconscious Mind communicating. Just encourage the client to feel the feeling. Show that it's safe to allow those feeling to be there. *You're* safe to feel those feelings with. There's no need to stuff anything down. It's okay to just let it out. Feelings are normal and natural. They're part of the human experience.

> For example, "Anyone who had been through what you've been through would feel the same way. You're allowed to feel (mad, sad, hurt, etc.) Those are your feelings. You're allowed to have all your feelings and heal. The truth is . . . you're not the first person to walk down that road. Sadly, you probably won't be the last. We're here to get you healed. We're here to get you free of the past so that you can feel good about yourself and move forward with your life. Understand?"

Make it safe for the client to face their truest feelings because you're going to be asking the client to *let you* guide them into the part of their Mind that has the Power to create the change they want. That takes trust. You're going to be asking the Subconscious Mind to show you what the Conscious Mind doesn't know, or doesn't *want* to know, can't fix, and in most cases, has been trying to avoid. That takes trust. You're going to be asking the Conscious Mind to allow uncomfortable feelings to come to awareness. That takes trust.

Regression Happens

When a client is feeling an emotion, they're already beginning to regress. They may not realize what's happening, but that feeling isn't coming out of what's happening now. It's coming out of a past event that has everything to do with that feeling. Remember, there's nothing going on in your office to cause the feeling. What's bubbling up to conscious awareness is coming out of an event in the past. But something just happened in your session to trigger a memory.

What happened? What was the client just talking about or remembering? Pay close attention to the words the client is using. Subtle shifts in language and tonality can indicate that the client has regressed to a younger age. For example, the client may speak more quietly or in a slightly higher voice. I had a client say, "touched my pee-pee." These are not the words of the Conscious, Adult, Thinking Mind. These are the words of the Child Mind. That's the Subconscious Mind communicating.

Memories and emotions are how the Subconscious Mind communicates. The client just needs to know that it's safe to let it communicate by reminding the client that they're allowed to feel the feeling. For example, "That feeling is allowed to be there. All your feelings are good – even the uncomfortable ones. You let yourself feel that feeling. Feeling the feeling releases the feeling so that you can feel better."

Emotion is nothing to be afraid of. Feelings naturally arise and pass away, provided we let ourselves feel them. What makes a feeling so uncomfortable is our resistance to feeling them. Avoidance doesn't get rid of the feeling. It just drives it further underground. Trying to avoid a feeling, or blocking its expression, only reinforces the problem by adding to the internal accumulation of unresolved emotional debris. When the pressure becomes too much to bear, the lid will come off. That's called abreaction.

Abreactions Happen

When a client abreacts, they are doing a deep dive into the Subconscious Mind. This can result in a spontaneous regression. What's happening is the Mind is associating back into a past event. The problem is that all you can see is what's happening on the surface. You may see a flush of strong emotion, but you'll have no idea what's happening on the inside. You have to ask. When you see an emotion flooding into consciousness, ask immediately, "What just happened?"

An abreaction is a natural and normal human experience. It's nothing to be afraid of. It's just that it happened very suddenly. It was unexpected. And there's a little more volume than the client is comfortable with. That's evidence that the client has been trying to keep a lid on that feeling for too long. What just happened? Nothing. The client had a thought. A picture came to mind. Something about that image triggered the feelings—a basic stimulus-response.

Pictures and images are connected to memories. That memory is of an event that over and done. The problem is that Subconscious Mind doesn't know this. The client got triggered and reacted *as if* they were still in that situation. This is essentially what a flashback is like. It's something from that past that, in the person's mind, is happening all over again.

When a client abreacts, the lid just popped off an undigested memory. Something about that event hasn't been brought to completion. It's still unresolved and, as a result, is still available for triggering. But when a client dives into an uncomfortable feeling and abreacts, they are handing you a gift. Honor the gift by honoring the feeling. Prove that you're not going to leave them stuck in an uncomfortable emotion by taking charge and proving to the client that they don't have to suppress their feelings. They don't have to avoid their feelings. They don't have to put a lid on how they feel. It's okay to feel a feeling. They won't die if they just feel it. Avoiding feelings and memories only makes things worse. This is why you should never try to suggest away an emotion.

The Subconscious Mind wants the same thing you do—for the client to be safe and feel better. It just doesn't have a choice. It must protect, and sometimes it will do so in ways we don't like. If you try to override the Subconscious Mind's Prime Directive, you won't get very far. You'll run into resistance, and the client will struggle unnecessarily. It's like trying to close the barn door when the horses are trying to bust free. If you do, you're likely to get hurt in the process.

Instead of trying to slam the door shut on an uncomfortable feeling, give it permission to express. All you need to do is take charge and direct the energy. Give it permission to be there. Then, give it a place to go. You can have the client tap it out or put it into a pillow. They can breathe through it or speak it out. Feeling the emotion is what releases it. That's what is going to help the client to feel better. Show the client how to safely move through an uncomfortable emotion. Prove that it's possible to feel better. Teach the client that it's okay to feel a feeling. *Just feel it.* All that's happening is some uncomfortable feelings are finding their way out. That's good.

Feelings naturally want to move, so any movement will help the client to feel better very quickly. As a result, they will discover that emotions don't last very long when they just let themselves feel the feeling. Even the worst feeling won't last more than ninety seconds if the client just feels it. Then, it's over. Most people don't know this. When an emotion starts to find its way to the surface of awareness, they slam the lid down. This keeps them stuck in a pattern of recycling the same thoughts and feelings, over and over, which reinforce the problem. As a result, the problem gets worse over time.

You can put an end to emotional recycling by stepping in and taking charge. This will empower the client to allow more feelings to come up and be expressed during the process, making your job easier. Best of all, the client will get what they most need—relief. That's healing.

How Strong Is It?

If the client is feeling a strong emotion, take a SUD to measure the intensity of the feeling. This will allow you to match the method of releasing to the intensity of the emotion. "On a scale of one to ten, how strong is that feeling?"

If the client's SUD is a five or six, talking is often enough to discharge the energy. Encourage the client to speak the truth of how they feel while feeling the feeling in the body. For example, "I feel sad." Or, "I feel angry!"

If the SUD is higher, you can invite the client to tap on it or pump the feeling into a pillow. A more intense emotion (10+) can give you a Bridge straight back into the ISE. The client is already halfway there. All you really need to do is just instruct the client to focus on the feeling and follow it back to an earlier event. Do that, and you'll make the client a believer. They'll realize that what caused them to feel that way has everything to do with a past experience. They'll understand how their own Mind has been holding onto that feeling, that it's there for a reason. This puts them back in choice.

Once the client understands what caused the problem, they won't have to continue to hold onto the feeling any longer. What an awesome liberating thing to discover. What a new sense of empowerment they can take home with them!

Freaking Out!

What if the client starts freaking out? What if it seems like the client is spiraling down? What if they're getting worse? The number one job is to provide safety. Get them out. If the client can't speak, if they're feeling overwhelmed, there may be a problem with the client's ability to manage their emotions.

Emotional dysregulation can be indicative of unresolved trauma. If the client is overwhelmed, realize it's too much for them. They don't feel in control. Somebody needs to be in control to protect the client. That somebody needs to be you. If you don't know what to do, or the abreaction takes you by surprise, or you're just not prepared for the intensity, the best thing to do is to just get the client out. Speak calmly and firmly. Tell them to open their eyes and look at you. Don't touch them. Just instruct them to focus on you and take a nice, deep breath in. As they follow your instructions, say, "That's right. Well, done."

Once the client has settled down and is breathing rhythmically, find out what just happened. You can then deal with it in retrospect by tapping on "what just happened." This will help to release the residual emotions attached to the memory. For example, "A moment ago I bumped into an uncomfortable feeling /And even though I was feeling (scared) / I'm okay now / I'm right here / Alive and well / going deeper.".

To process "what just happened" work in past tense. This allows the client to get some emotional distance from whatever was freaking them out while you help them to release the charge. The client's resistance to the feeling is 90% of the problem. Teach your clients that it's safe to feel their feelings. Feeling the feeling releases the feeling. Releasing the feeling allows them to feel better. As soon as they notice a shift toward the better, acknowledge it. Validating every positive shift and every movement toward a better feeling will help the client to feel more in control and, therefore, more ready to face the event from the past that generated that uncomfortable feeling.

If the client opens their eyes and they're still freaking out, realize they're stuck in a memory. You need to take charge by using an authoritarian tone to bring them back into the here and now. Ask questions that help the client to associate into present time and space. For example: "What day is this? / Where are you right now? / What time is it?"

The client won't be able to think until you get them calmed down, so wait until they're fully present and can pay attention to you. Then help them to realize three important truths. First, they're okay. Second, they're not alone. Third, you know what to do. Help your clients to understand that their Subconscious Mind is designed to take care of them.

Ditch the Script

They need to know there's nothing wrong with them, that their Subconscious is doing exactly what it was designed to do. Their Subconscious just stepped in to avoid a *perceived* threat. Because the Subconscious Mind cannot distinguish between a real and an imagined threat, it responded *as if* it were real. The Subconscious Mind doesn't realize the client isn't in that past situation anymore. As far as it's concerned, it's all still happening now.

Anything you can do to get the client to participate in bringing the energy intensity down is going to be empowering for the client. You can tap through the thoughts and feelings the client is experiencing. You can have them simply tap on the karate chop point or rub the "sore spots" on the upper chest while stating out loud, "I feel (insert emotion)." This validates the feeling. Alternately, you could have them rub or tap on the collar bone points. All are effective at helping to calm the nervous system of the body.

Use Autosuggestion

If you don't yet know tapping, just use autosuggestion. It's very effective because the client is participating in their own healing. When the client makes a statement about themselves, to themselves, it has more power than anything you might suggest to them. Use autosuggestion to help restore balance by having the client repeat positive suggestions that reinforce the truth. For example: "I'm okay. / I'm still here. / I'm safe now. / I know I'm okay because (put an ending on it)."

Keep at it until the client calms down. Once the client is breathing more rhythmically, you can use a retrospective approach to process what just happened. Something just happened to trigger them, but you have no idea what that might be. Where did their Mind just take them? You need to find out. Then you can process that memory in hindsight. The way to do this is by using past-tense language to acknowledge what just happened. For example, "I was thinking about (this) / and it made me feel (emotion, i.e., okay) / And NOW I feel (emotion, I.e., okay) . . ."

This helps the client recognize that something happened to trigger the emotional response. Usually, it was a thought. Help the client make the connection between *that* thought and *that* feeling. This helps the client to take responsibility for their own thoughts and feelings. Remember, it's their Mind. For example, "Even though a moment ago I had the thought (I'm going to die), and it makes me feel (scared), I'm okay *now*." This brings them back into the present moment more fully. Once they accept that they're okay, they'll feel more in control.

Recognize that when a client abreacts, this is the Subconscious Mind expressing a need for safety. It's doing exactly what it was designed to do—keep the client safe by avoiding threats. The fact that the threat is in the past hasn't registered yet. That's the purpose of the regression work—put the past in the past. You can guide the client through a series of statements that affirm that they're safe because the event is in the past. For example, "I'm okay. / It's in the past. / I made it through. / I'm safe now. / So, I can relax."

Reframe

It's not what just happened that's the problem. It's that the client is judging themselves for losing control. They're feeling a bit crazy because they don't know what just happened. It came out of nowhere. That just adds to the anxiety they're already feeling. Identify these thoughts and clear them. When your client realizes they're okay, you can reframe what just happened in a positive light. Use it as evidence that their Subconscious Mind really wants to get this problem resolved. Let them know they're in the perfect place to do that. This will help the client to realize that they are, in fact, creating this response and that its' possible to feel better.

If You're freaking out . . .

What do you do if the client starts freaking out and *you* start freaking out? If it feels like it's too much for *you*, it probably is. Keep your focus on the client. Your primary responsibility is always to the client. If you're feeling overwhelmed, get the client out by giving the instruction, "The scene fades and you grow peaceful with your breathing." Then, emerge the client. Bring their attention back fully to the present moment. When a person emerges from hypnosis, they're still hyper-suggestible. Keep pouring in suggestions to help the client re-stabilize.

Slow their breathing down by guiding them to extend the outbreath just a little. Using a count can help keep to keep the client focused on your voice. For example, "Nice deep breath in, one, two, three, that's right. And now exhale, one, two, three, four. Very good. You're here now, doing fine. One more time." Repeat until the client is breathing normally.

Realize the client is probably feeling like a crazy person. Reassure them that this is just how the Mind works, they just bumped into an uncomfortable memory, it's *only* a memory, and they're safe, all grown up, here with you now. Let them talk about their experience in hindsight. Do a little reframing. Then, consider referring the client out to an appropriate mental healthcare worker. Remember, you need clients you can be successful with, not clients who are going to dump you into the deep end with sharks!

Time Investment

I prefer to complete the intake process before guiding the client into a past event because regression can take time. Before we start diving into painful past events, I want to teach the client how to be successful working with me. This can save you time when you most need it. If the client bumps into a strong emotion during the intake, you can use it as an opportunity to teach the client how to honor their feelings.

Teach them how to feel better by releasing uncomfortable feelings and emotions. The client will discover just how quickly they can feel better, and their feelings won't have such a hold over them. Not only will this give you a client who is willing to trust you to guide them where they need to go to get the healing, but they'll also be less fearful of facing their feelings when confronted by them. This will give you a much more resourceful client to do the work when you start guiding them through the process of Regression to Cause.

The hypnosis profession has been too quick to toss out the therapeutic value of giving the client permission to speak prior to the induction. We don't want to be accused of practicing "talk therapy." And for good reason. Talk alone won't solve the client's issue. Telling the same

Story, over and over again, may provide some temporary relief. It may even result in a few insights into the cause of the problem. But it doesn't *change* anything.

Talking may discharge some of the energy in the Story, but the person still has the problem. As a result, the energy tends to build back up, again, putting the client on a hamster wheel of ongoing therapy. You don't want to be "that guy." While Regression Hypnotherapy is considered a brief therapy, it's not a quick fix. Its effectiveness lies in working with the part of the Mind that has the power to create real and lasting change. The time it takes is really up to the client. Your intake is an investment of time that allows you to demonstrate that you can be trusted, that you're safe. Listening to the client's Pain Story is a way to earn the cooperation of both the Conscious Mind and the Subconscious Mind so that they'll *let* you guide the process. This is what your intake process can give you. It isn't merely a brief introduction before guiding the client into hypnosis. It's an interactive process where you're establishing rapport with both the Conscious and Subconscious levels of Mind.

Healing isn't something you do. Healing is something that happens when the client is ready to *let* it happen. Your job is simply to create the conditions where it's safe to allow healing to happen. This is what you are setting up for. Sometimes, it's enough to just prove that it's okay to feel a feeling. Sometimes it's enough to show the client that it's safe to face their history, that it's possible to heal. Sometimes, it's everything.

Summary

The intake process is not merely a conversation. It's a strategy for establishing the Therapeutic Relationship while you assess the client's readiness to proceed with you. If you listen carefully, the client will give you everything you need to guide the healing process effectively.

The intake is the first step in the client's healing process. This is where you listen to the Conscious Mind's Pain Story to gain the cooperation of both the Conscious and Subconscious Mind. When you take on the role of guide and protector, the Conscious Mind will be less inclined to try to run the show, and the Subconscious Mind will relax and work with you.

The purpose of the intake process is to establish a Therapeutic Relationship in which it is safe for the client to face their deepest, darkest secrets so that they can heal. The Therapeutic Relationship provides a safe place for healing to happen. Your intake allows you to gather up the information you need to chart a course to the client's goal while making it safe for your client to accept your suggestions.

The client needs to feel safe with you before you start delivering suggestions because everything you do in a hypnosis session is based on suggestion. Hypnosis happens through suggestion. Regression happens through suggestion. Change happens when a suggestion is accepted. And the client is always choosing, either consciously or unconsciously, whether or not to accept your suggestions based on their level of trust.

The intake is also a process of laying the foundation for the Therapeutic Contract. The Therapeutic Contract gives you permission to guide the healing process. The information you gather during the intake allows you to customize your educational pre-talk to the specific needs and concerns of each client. During the intake process, you can help your client to safely connect with painful emotions that have everything to do with their presenting issue. This gives the Subconscious Mind permission to tell its Story. You can then teach the client how to safely release a feeling to feel better.

Hypnosis happens. When a client is feeling an emotion, they are already in hypnosis. The stronger the emotion, the deeper the hypnosis. When you have deep hypnosis, regression happens. When you have a highly emotional client or someone who is deeply distressed, it's usually because the problem has been around for a while. They have a history with that problem. That's where the internal pressure is coming from. This can result in a spontaneous regression or abreaction.

An abreaction is a gift. You can use it to Bridge back to the event that caused it or teach the client how to release some of the internal pressure to feel better. This teaches the client that it's possible to feel better very quickly.

You can learn more about my approach to the first session in the Ready for Regression First Session System course here: https://www.tribeofhealers.com/ready-for-regression-first-session-system-course/

CHAPTER 5:
Intake Assessments

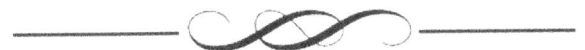

During the intake process, you are uncovering the client's Pain Story. You are validating the feelings in the Story and showing the Subconscious Mind that you can be trusted to honor how it feels. This is why it is important not to rush the client during the intake. It's because the Subconscious Mind is the Feeling Mind, and the feeling Mind is the Child Mind. Children are often bullied into hurrying up and doing as they're told. This just creates resistance. That won't help you when it comes time to do the hypnosis.

You want to set things up so well that the client will automatically take the next step. Then, it becomes a natural process of guiding the client step by step right out of the problem. Listening and observing the client's responses during the intake process will allow you to assess the client's readiness to proceed with the healing process.

Assess Rapport

I'm not an advocate for dumping people into their stuff. People are coming to you because they've been traumatized. Respect the Subconscious Mind's need to protect. If the client seems to be holding back, there's a reason. This may indicate where the healing process needs to begin – proving that it's safe for the client to let you do your job. For example, if the client is apprehensive about the hypnosis, find out what their specific concerns are so that you can educate them in a way that makes it safe to trust you.

During the intake, pay attention to how the client is responding to you during the intake to gauge your level of rapport. Are they forthcoming? Or do they seem to be holding back? If the client doesn't trust you, they won't be willing to let you guide the process.

Assess Verbal and Non-Verbal Responses

During the process, pay careful attention to both verbal and non-verbal communication in response to the intake questions. For example, what does the client's body posture suggest? Are you noticing some tension in the body? What are the client's emotional responses? Is there too much feeling present or too little? Does the client use metaphor to describe how they feel? How emotionally literate is the client? Do they use thinking to override feeling? Do they use thinking words like "rejected," "stressed," "upset," "anxious," "overwhelmed," and "depressed" instead of emotional words like "sad," "scared," or "angry"?

Words have power. The client may *think* they're feeling stressed when, in fact, they're feeling sad. They may think they're feeling upset when, in fact, they're feeling scared. They may think they're feeling anxious when, in fact, they're feeling angry. Words like "upset" or "overwhelmed" refer to an emotional experience but they're not the emotion. As a result, they create distance from what the client is actually feeling. When it comes to emotional healing work, the more specific you can be with your language, the better your results will be. You won't know what the client's Subconscious Mind is trying to communicate until the client names the emotion. To identify the actual emotion, ask the client, "If that (stressed) feeling could speak, what would it say?" or "If that (betrayed) feeling was an emotion, what would it be – mad, sad, scared or something else?" Grind down to the Subconscious truth. That's the feeling.

Assess Emotional Stability

How emotionally stable is the client? If your client is coming emotionally undone, that's okay. Feelings and emotions are the territories in which you work. But if it feels like it's too much for *you*, you might want to consider referring them out to someone more experienced. Some people can be a bit of a handful in the session room. The last thing you need is a client who is going to throw you into the deep end . . . with sharks.

Assess Emotional Connectivity

Candace Pert, the author of *Molecules of Emotion*, stated, "Your body is your Subconscious Mind." That's where we feel our feelings—in the body. Emotions are Subconscious communication that is felt physically in the body. Emotions are felt in targeted areas of the body, primarily in the gut, chest, or throat. "That fear" in the gut. "That sadness" in the chest. "That anger" in the throat. These are specific emotional signals that are tied to specific events in the client's past.

To feel fully alive requires emotional connectivity. Unfortunately, many people learn early in life to disconnect from their feelings and emotions. This may have been a necessary survival strategy in childhood, but it disconnects a person from themselves. This is a very common pattern with people suffering from depression. They learned to avoid their feelings. The emotions are still there. But instead of allowing their emotions to come to awareness to be expressed, the person pushes them back down, keeping the feelings bottled up inside.

If your client habitually disconnects from their emotional body, they may find it difficult to find a feeling. This can make it more difficult to find a Bridge to the Past. Teaching your client how to find a feeling can make it much easier to locate the cause of the emotion and release it. You can use the following exercise, adapted from Eugene Gendlin's book, *Focusing*, to teach a client how to find and feel a feeling in the body. First, instruct the client to close their eyes, go inside, and follow your instructions. Then guide them through the following series of experiences.

Felt-Sense Exercise

> Focus on your big toe. Wiggle it a little. Press it down. Notice how that feels. When you have a sense of that, let me know. (Wait for a response.)
>
> Notice the sensations inside your big toe. Notice what that feels like. When you have a sense of that, let me know. (This might take them a few moments, so just wait quietly. Let the client be responsible for the results!)
>
> Bring your awareness up the leg to the knee. Notice the feeling of sensation of the knee. For example, the position of the knee or anything that might be touching the knee. Then find the feeling inside the knee. When you have that, let me know. (Wait for a response.)
>
> Come up to the groin and into the stomach. (When they notice the feeling inside the stomach, you're there!)
>
> Come up further into the chest, sense what's there.
>
> Come up into the throat. Notice the feeling and sensations there.

And you're done! You have now successfully associated the client into their body. This is just one simple strategy you can use to quickly help a client to reconnect with their ability to feel their feelings. This may seem like such a small thing, but you are actually helping the client to reconnect with a Part of themselves that they have been closed off from. When it comes time to do the regression work, it can end the frustration of trying to find emotion—for both you and your client.

The trick is to make the client responsible for the result. It should only take a few seconds for the client to notice a sensation in the body. If they can't find the feeling, they're just not paying close enough attention to what's happening in the body. That's the underlying problem. The client has learned to avoid awareness of their feelings. That's got to stop!

Changing this self-destructive pattern begins right here by requiring the client to pay attention to feelings and emotions. It's also a cornerstone of the Therapeutic Contract. The client must agree to follow your instructions. Be patient. Give the client the time they need to successfully find the feeling. The only people who can't feel anything are dead. The client just needs to learn how to *notice* their feelings.

Nothing builds success like success. The moment the client notices a feeling or sensation in the body, celebrate success. Validate it by saying, "Good job!" Or, "That's right!" Or, "Now you've got it." This teaches the client to associate success with allowing feelings and sensations to come to awareness. This teaches the client that it's safe to let their Subconscious Mind communicate.

Some clients are mentally scattered. Sometimes, this is due to anxiety. Sometimes, it's a side-effect of medications. Sometimes, it's because they're in dire need of sleep. Chronic sleep deprivation leaves them feeling exhausted and unable to cope with daily living. You can improve a person's life dramatically simply by helping them to sleep better.

Just getting enough rest will help to improve how the client feels about themselves and others and brighten their general outlook on life. Helping your clients to sleep better will also give you a better client to work with because lack of sleep messes with cognition. It's the leading cause of accidents, both on the road and in the workplace. Improving the quality of your client's sleep will give you a more insightful and attentive participant in the healing process.

If your client seems to be really scattered or spinney, it might be helpful to begin the healing process by teaching them some grounding exercises. Getting them out of their head and into their body will give you a much better client to work with.

Grounding Exercise

Invite the client to close their eyes and go inside the body and imagine . . . what it might be like . . . to have roots . . . growing out of the bottoms of their feet. Then, send those roots down into the earth, through all the layers of the earth, all the way down into the very core of the planet.

Invite the client to describe what they find there. What do they discover at the core of the planet? Does it have a color? A temperature? A vibrational quality? What does it feel like? (Most often, the color is either red or gold.) Instruct the client to tap into this vital energy and draw it up, thirstily, through their roots. Draw it up-up-up into the bottoms of the feet. And now you are all set up for a reverse progressive relaxation!

Draw the energy up into the feet and the calves; notice how that feels. Move progressively up through the body to the top of the head. Then, send it back down throughout the body, from the top of the head to the bottoms of the feet, relaxing every muscle, nerve, and fiber of the body. It feels so good! Finally, offer the suggestion that the client can use this imagery exercise anything time they want or need to feel more grounded and relaxed.

This exercise doesn't require hypnosis. Once learned, it only takes a few minutes to put down roots and draw the energy up into the nervous system of the body. I use it before I go shopping at Costco. It works like a hot damn!

Assess Expectations

Some people think that they're going to lie back, have a nap, and emerge from hypnosis transformed. That's not hypnosis. It's magic. We've all been to a pill for every ill. The client is not difficult. It's just what they learned. The problem is that the "fix me" expectation won't get them what they need. It's not like they're dropping the car off to get the brakes fixed. That old model of the mind as a machine is not only outdated, but it also contributes to shame, and vulnerability, and dependency. We want to put an end to those things but to do that requires the client's participation. You need a client who is willing to take responsibility for doing their own work because you can't do it for them.

Your job isn't to figure anything out. Your job is to ask the Subconscious Mind to show you what's needed to resolve the problem. Then you can find a way to provide it. How willing is the client to participate in their own healing?

Summary

Throughout the intake process, you can be listening, observing, and assessing the client's readiness for regression by paying attention to the following factors.

- What is the client's level of rapport?
- What information is being communicated verbally?
- What are the client's non-verbal responses telling you?
- How emotionally stable is the client?
- How in touch is the client with their feelings and emotions?
- Is the client mentally scattered?
- Are the client's quality and quantity of sleep an issue?
- How willing is the client to participate in their own healing process?

Surface techniques like direct suggestion and guided imagery are suitable for managing symptoms. They're effective at providing comfort or helping a person to cope. For example, a person undergoing medical treatment, receiving chemotherapy, or preparing for the end of life can be treated with surface techniques. But when it comes to emotional issues, a person can't simply imagine themselves into a better belief. – **The Devil's Therapy**

CHAPTER 6:
Symptom Resolution Keys

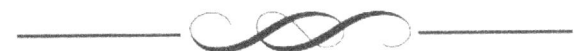

Every problem a person brings to you has roots in a past experience. This means that the client's issue is unique to their personal history. You won't know what the *real* problem is until their Subconscious Mind shows you. The Subconscious Mind's side of the client's issue is the emotional Story. This will be revealed through the healing process. What it will show you is how the client's problem got started and how the problem developed over time.

What it won't tell you is the facts about what happened. This is because the Subconscious Mind's Story doesn't keep a record of truth or fact. It stores a record of the perceptions, thoughts, and feelings that made an impression at the time an event occurred. All the Subconscious Mind can show you is how the client interpreted a specific situation and how it made them feel. That's what needs to change.

You can't change a person's past. Whatever happened to cause the problem is ancient history. It's over. What you can change is how the client thinks about past events that caused them pain. This will change how they feel.

Feelings drive behavior and responses to situations in daily life that find expression as unwanted symptoms. Changing how the client feels will change how the client responds to situations in daily life – mentally, physically, and emotionally.

The following ten Strategic Intake Questions can help you to begin the process of uncovering the information you need to locate and resolve the root cause of the client's problem. While you are guiding the client through this process, the key is keeping the focus on feelings and emotions.

1. *What is the problem?*

Emotional problems come in two flavors—Simple and Complex. Simple issues are rooted in a single event and are relatively simple to resolve. A simple issue usually has a single root-cause event that once resolved, removes the requirement for symptom expression. Often, the cause is based on the misperceptions of the Child. What was happening during the event was misinterpreted, causing the Child distress. This is the basic model most of us were taught in hypnosis school.

Bringing Adult Consciousness into the event can quickly resolve any misunderstandings to restore internal harmony. But not always. An experience of rape may be a one-time event, but it involves intense emotions. When there's a significant emotional charge trapped in an event, there can be multiple layers of perceptions, thoughts, and feelings that can take time to clear. A one-time, big-bang event early in life can also impact identity. It can shape how a person sees themselves as a result of that experience. Because of the tendency of the Subconscious Mind to generalize all learning, this can have a widespread effect on the client's life. For example, birth trauma can impact a person dramatically for the rest of their life.

Simple Issues

Simple Issues involve one ISE. This seeds the problem. Subsequent situations later in life then act as reminders of the causal event, restimulating the underlying pattern, and making it stronger. This repetitive reinforcement of the pattern means that, over time, the internal pressure is building up. As a result, things get worse. This is called the Compounding Effect. The Subconscious Mind naturally reinforces all learning. For this reason, Regression Hypnotherapy focuses on locating the ISE.

Do you have to find the ISE? No. It's simply easier to deal with a problem at its inception. It hasn't had time to grow and develop into a major problem yet. Trying to resolve a lifetime of accumulated thought and emotional energies can be hard work for both you and the client. Because the ISE is the first time the client experienced the feeling that is generating the symptoms, that event will have the weakest emotional charge attached to it, making it much easier to process. Simple, right?

Complex Issues

Complex Issues are another story. Complex issues aren't just one thing. They involve multiplicity. For example, a person facing the threat of diagnosis may be suffering from depression or feelings of fear, frustration and anger piled up on top of the primary problem. Complex issues can take more time to resolve completely

The Subconscious Mind is very specific. While a specific symptom will be formed as a result of a specific experience, there can be multiple ISEs, each requiring different symptoms or responses based on the specific impressions made by the event.

There can also be multiple events feeding into the problem. Different events can share the same theme while contributing different aspects to the client's symptoms. There can also be more than one offender contributing to the client's issue.

There can be multiple experiences within a single event generating multiple emotions expressing through symptoms. Think layers. To get a complete resolution of the problem, you have to uncover the layers of perceptions, thoughts, and feelings trapped in the event.

Trauma

Trauma comes in two sizes—big and little. Big trauma is the obvious stuff – rape, witnessing a murder, surviving a plane crash. Little trauma is the stuff that most people overlook because, to Adult Consciousness, it seems like no big deal. But to a Child, small things can feel overwhelming. That's what trauma is. It's an experience of overwhelm. It's not what happened that's the problem, however. It's how what was happening was being interpreted at that time.

Trauma has been defined as the perception of threat while in a state of helplessness. The keyword here is "perception." Human beings take in information through five sensory perception channels. We see, we hear, we smell, we taste, and we feel. We then evaluate these perceptions. Most of the time, this is an Unconscious process. The most basic evaluation is for safety. "Is this safe?" That's the Subconscious Mind's primary concern – safety – because safety serves survival.

A child is dependent on others to provide safety. If the Child has to deal with a scary situation alone, or is unable to make sense of what's happening, or lacks the ability to take action to protect himself, the Subconscious Mind is going to generate a distress signal called fear. The threat doesn't even have to be real. An imagined threat will generate real fear. For example, if Mom and Dad having an argument will generate real fear in the Child. A Child being dropped off at daycare for the first time can interpret the experience as abandonment. That's a very real threat to survival.

Problems that are rooted very early in life impact brain development and identity. When there are lots of recurring events early in life, neural pathways become like wagon ruts. With every repetition, the rut gets deeper. These deeply rooted patterns can take time to re-route simply because they have been reinforced from the earliest age. For example, childhood abuse is seldom a one-time event. It always generates confusion, fear, and anger. If the abuse was at the hands of a loved one, there's betrayal and a loss of trust. But all the emotions get mixed up with love. That's complexity.

Alcoholism in the family system means that the Child is growing up in a toxic environment where it's impossible to predict another's behavior. An alcoholic can be happy and loving one moment and raging out of control the next. This generates anxiety and confusion. Often, it develops an inability to trust one's own perceptions. The same is true of growing up with a mentally ill person, having to endure neglect, and surviving physical, mental, and sexual abuse.

If you have a client who is living with an alcoholic or an abusive spouse, they're not stuck in a bad situation. They're choosing to remain there because discomfort is their Comfort Zone. Choosing to remain in a toxic environment is not a conscious choice. It's a by-product of the client's history. On some level, their current environment is acceptable because, Subconsciously, it's familiar. A client who is going through bankruptcy or divorce, dealing with interpersonal conflicts at home or at work, or undergoing litigation, isn't just dealing with the present-day stressors. They're swimming against an undertow of past emotional events that resonate with the present situation. The added stress just makes them more vulnerable to getting triggered.

You can use all these things to resolve the client's presenting issue. Just keep in mind that while you strive to move them into more peaceful waters, you'll need to button up[3] the client for the period between sessions. Sometimes, progress will be two steps forward and one step back because, to achieve a complete resolution of the problem, you need to clear all the aspects contributing to the client's issue. This is the secret to working with complex issues – persist. Thoroughly release everything, and there will be nothing left to generate the symptoms.

Syndromes

When a client presents with multiple symptoms, you're not dealing with a single issue. You're dealing with a syndrome. A syndrome isn't just one thing. It's a cluster of symptoms all working together to create a pattern. The pattern is then given a name. For example, fibromyalgia is

---

[3] This is a term Stephen Parkhill used to refer to wrapping up a session when the healing process has not yet been completed. Buttoning up the client/session is like closing the wound, temporarily, so that you can come back later to finish the job.

a syndrome. Chronic fatigue is a syndrome. Syndromes often show up in your office in the form of a diagnosis. But if you try to treat the diagnosis, you won't get anywhere because the diagnosis is just a label required by a physician to prescribe treatment. You can't fix a label. Depression is a label. If you try to treat depression, you'll get nowhere. You need to find out how the client is "doing" depression. Then you can address each of the contributing aspects.

When you're dealing with a syndrome, your best strategy is to identify each individual symptom and deal with it separately. Make a list of all the symptoms that are contributing to the problem. How does the client know there even is a problem? Where does it hurt? How does the problem express? Once you have a list of all the symptoms, you can systematically "undo" them, one by one. This is the key to resolving the client's issue - focus on one thing at a time. One goal. One symptom. One thought. One feeling. This will give you a clearer path to the cause and a much more thorough clearing of the contributing aspects. If you're lucky, all the symptoms will be rooted in a single event making it a simple issue to resolve.

The Snowball Effect

Like most problems, a syndrome starts out as one problem. Because its unresolved, other problems get added to the pattern over time. There's a snowball effect. The problem may have started out as something small in the ISE, but it has continued to grow and develop through Subsequent Sensitizing Events (SSEs), adding more aspects to the pattern. This adds complexity. The more recurrence of events there are, the more reinforcement of the underlying pattern occurs, and the more stuff gets added to the snowball as it bounces through childhood. As a result, the more recent symptoms will tend to be more painful or distressing, motivating the person to seek help.

2. *When did the problem begin?*

When did the symptoms first appear? When did the unwanted behavior get started? The causal event is going to be some time before then. Find out when the client first noticed symptoms coming on. Usually, it starts with one thing—for example, headaches. Then something else added to it. It's like a snowball rolling downhill, picking up stuff as it picks up speed. You'll find this with smoking clients. The habit didn't start with the first cigarette. That's just when the Subconscious Mind found a way to meet a need by using cigarettes. The behavior is just a symptom of the unmet need. What you're looking for is a Bridge to regress back further on. What feeling motivated the client to put the cigarette in their mouth? Focus on that feeling!

What caused the person to put that first cigarette in their mouth happened long before they lit up. The first cigarette is not the causal event. It's the Symptom Producing Event (SPE). If the client can identify the earliest symptom, it can give you a good place to start the regression because it's a shorter Bridge back to the causal event. This can save time in session because all you need to do is go back to when that specific symptom first appeared – the ache, the pain, the lump, the bump, or the first cigarette. Uncover the circumstances associated with the specific symptom. Bring up the feeling associated with that event and start Bridging back to locate the earliest event. The earliest event is the causal event. It's the first time. Resolve what's there, then see what's left.

People with serious illnesses usually have a history of lesser ailments. This is another function of your intake process. If you're dealing with a medical issue, have a look at the client's health history. The first symptom that came on is usually something minor, so the client won't realize there's a connection to their presenting issue. Small things like eczema, asthma, or allergies in childhood may seem unrelated, but you'll discover they're part of a larger story when you start doing the regression work.

A consciously remembered event is rarely the causal event, but if you can identify a specific consciously-remembered event, it gives you a place to begin the regression. This can save you session time because the causal event will be prior to the consciously remembered event. For example, if the client says the problem started when he was a four-year-old, you know the causal event will be some time before the age of four.

During the intake, find out what was happening in the client's life at that time. What was going on in the family system at that time? How were Mom and Dad getting along? Were there any siblings? Watch for clues such as substance abuse, divorce, the birth of a new baby into the family system. See if you can identify a specific event that might have triggered the symptoms to first appear. This gives you a starting point for the regression.

Nobody gets cancer first. – Stephen Parkhill

Hypnosis enhances recall so, once you get the client into hypnosis, you'll have access to more of the details. Once you have deepened to somnambulism, you can direct the client to go back to the consciously remembered event, and you're all set up for the regression. Reviewing the event will help to deepen the hypnosis while allowing you to find a Bridge.

Most problems start out small and get bigger over time. This means that the first consciously remembered event will be a lower intensity than a more recent event. The ISE will be lower, still. But what if you're dealing with a client who has panic attacks? You don't want to guide the client back into a panic attack. That's unnecessary. But everyone remembers the first time they had a panic attack. That's all the information you need to begin the regression.

When you guide the client back into the consciously remembered event, instruct them to go back *before* anything has happened. Ensure that you are taking the client back to a moment when she's still feeling safe and secure. Rule number one is safety. The client does not have to relive a panic attack! You just need to find out what happens just before the panicky feeling comes on. One moment the client will be feeling fine, then something will happen to change that. What happens? When does the feeling change from okay to something else? What happens to trigger that feeling?

The answer lies in how the client is perceiving what's happening in the event. What is he seeing? Hearing? Smelling? Touching? What's the trigger for "that feeling"? For example, the smell of cigarettes on his breath. Don't stop there. Find out how the client is interpreting that perception. What meaning is being assigned to that perception?

Sentence Stems Completion

Stems Completion Sentence is a valuable uncovering tool. You can use it to peel away the layers of perception, thought, and feeling to identify the underlying cause of the problem. For example, "The smell of cigarettes on his breath makes me think (put an ending on it.)."

That thought, whatever it is, is connected to an emotion. What emotion is it? Fear? Anger? Sadness? For example, let's say the client says, "The smell of cigarettes makes me think he's going to hurt me." Here, you would offer another Stems Completion Sentence to uncover the emotion being created by that thought, "The thought he's going to hurt me makes me feel (put an ending on it)."

Let's say that the client responds, ". . . scared!" You have just identified the Symptom Pattern. The perception (smell of breath) is being interpreted as a threat (the thought), which is generating the emotion of fear. You now have a Bridge to the event that caused that specific fear. Nice, right?

Here's another example. Let's say you're dealing with a compulsive eating problem. There's a moment where the craving starts to come on. "That feeling" is what motivates the client to dive into the bag of Doritos or seek solace in the Häagen-Dazs. That's the feeling you're looking for, the one that drives the out-of-control behavior.

It may not seem like a panic attack is a behavior, but it's a response to an uncomfortable emotion, in the same way, going face-first into the ice cream is a response to a feeling. The behavior is what happens when the client can't get away from the feeling. The purpose of the second question is to find out how the client first knew there even was a problem. How did the problem first present? How was it expressing? Because it may be different now. If you can identify what the first symptoms to express were, you can go "upstream" of how the problem is currently expressing. Resolve that earliest symptom, and you may just pull the plug on the whole pattern.

3. What else have you tried?

My physiotherapist says, "If you don't listen to the whispers, you'll have to put up with the shouts." Most of the people who show up in your office have been putting up with the shouts. The problem has been building up steam at a Subconscious level of Mind, and they just can't ignore the feeling anymore. If the client has been struggling with the problem for some time, they have probably tried other solutions before seeking out your help. The purpose of the third question is to dispel any doubts or fears regarding the process. These concerns may seem like small, niggling doubts or fears, but they have the power to block you. Find out what the client tried. What worked and didn't work? The client just needs to know how what you're offering is going to be any different. Then they can expect a different result.

Maybe what they tried didn't completely resolve the problem, but maybe it helped. If previous therapies helped at all, it's probably because they took off some of the surface layers. It's just that the client needs a deeper technique to resolve the problem for good. For example, I've found that clients who have been for counseling or psychotherapy are the best clients. They're not expecting you to wave your magic wand. They're highly motivated to heal. They're prepared to participate in the healing process, and they tend to be more self-aware and insightful.

Never disrespect the client's previous therapies. Empower your clients to trust themselves and their ability to make good decisions on their own behalf. Validate everything that they've done so far. Instill hope. Remind them that they're just not done yet. In fact, they could be inches from the finish line and not even realize it. Sometimes, you can find a way to build on the client's past experiences of success by using things that the client found helpful. For example, if a certain eating plan worked for the client in the past, show them how you can empower them to stick to a program by addressing the internal drive to overeat. You're not here to make them do anything. You're here to help them get back their power to choose. That's huge.

Past Failures

If previous attempts to solve the problem failed, the client is going to have feelings about that. It might be frustration. It might be anger. It might be guilt. For example, if the client has been through the medical mill, they've been sensitized to being poked and prodded and treated as a problem, not a person. These clients have a real need to feel that they're being heard. If the client is still angry with their last healing practitioner, they could subconsciously project that anger onto you. That will only get in your way. But if you ask them to tell you about it and then listen to what they've been through, you can show that you understand. You then become a trusted friend and confidant.

If something didn't work, it's simple. Let the client know that you're not going to do that. Whatever it was, find out what the client didn't like about it so that you'll know what to do differently. For example, if their last therapist tried a progressive relaxation induction, and they didn't like it, or they didn't get the results they wanted, don't do that! Use a different induction. Prove that what you do is different, and the client will expect a different result.

Resistance to the Technique

Some clients are resistant to regression. They'll say, "I don't want to go there." Obviously, you need to resolve that. Find out *why* they don't want to go there. You can then address this resistance during your educational pre-talk. You cannot allow the client to dictate the therapy. If you do, you're sunk. You need compliance to get the results. Compliance means cooperation. You need the client to be a willing participant in the healing process to be successful. To get the results, the client must be willing to go where you need them to go.

When there's resistance, there's always a reason.

I met a person who adamantly refused to even consider regression. Period. Not going there. Not open for discussion. I didn't try to argue with her. I just asked her, "How come?" In her case, she had good reason for wanting to avoid regression. She had been seeing a psychologist to work on an unresolved issue from her past. Her psychologist decided to try hypnosis with her. The client regressed to an experience of being raped.

Having to relive an experience of violence retraumatized her. No wonder she didn't want to go there! I won her trust by validating how she felt. I then explained why something like that could never happen in my office. Her psychologist may be licensed to practice psychotherapy, but he was clearly not qualified to facilitate Regression Hypnotherapy. If he was, he would have known what to do. The client's safety always comes first.

She agreed to become my client, provided I promise not to regress her into a painful event. I kept my promise. But I did regress her into a past event. I encouraged her to revivify it powerfully, too. This was an experience of sublime bliss while the client was sailing. She felt free and alive and completely connected to the Power of Nature. It was an amazing experience for both of us. I grabbed the opportunity to use a powerful resource state to help her overcome a major block in her life. Not only did this resolve the client's presenting issue, but it also restored her faith in therapy.

I've had clients who didn't want to do tapping. They'd tried it and "it didn't work." In every case, the client had tried Emotional Freedom Tapping (EFT) with their counselor or a psychologist. I cannot be held accountable for another therapist's lack of skill, so I just said, "Yah, I hear that a lot. This is different." I then asked the client to "treat it like cornflakes and try it again for the first time." With the client's permission, I then proved that what I do is different. That's all you need to do. Make it safe for the client to do what you're asking them to do. Prove that what you do is different. Show that you can help the client get some relief and you won't have a problem with compliance.

What about now?

Another question to ask the client is what, if anything, are they doing now? Some clients are undergoing medical treatment or working with other therapists. It's important to the client that you support these things. Whatever they're doing, use it. Empower your client's faith in their choices for healing because this supports them in healing. If the client has some kind of self-healing practice like yoga or meditation, this is a client who is willing to do their own work. The best clients are those who are willing to participate in their own healing. For example, I had a client who took up yoga. She loved it, so I asked her what she loved about it. She described how good it made her feel. When a client taps into some good feelings, make note! This is the stuff you can use to fill the client's tank during your Session Wrap Up. Just throw in a few suggestions at the end of each session to remind the client of what it's like to be in a state of love. Love heals.

If the client is receiving another source of care, sometimes a multi-pronged approach is what's needed to get a complete resolution of the problem. For example, I had a client with a serious snake phobia. She had already been through conventional therapies like Cognitive Behavioral Therapy (CBT) which helped her to cope with the problem. The problem was that she still had the problem. The client made marked progress with Regression Hypnotherapy, but she still had some niggling bit of resistance that just wouldn't let go. In reviewing her progress, the client revealed that she had been diagnosed with an organic issue that was directly connected to the autonomic nervous system. She informed me that this condition could well be contributing to her irrational fear. We agreed that it might be the right time for her to consult with her naturopath about the organic issue. This turned out to be very helpful and gave the client an added level of support in healing.

A cancer client, who refused to go the medical route and subject herself to chemotherapy, chose to work with a naturopath and a regression hypnotherapist instead. She received Vitamin C, intravenous (IV) treatments to boost her immune system while we worked on identifying and resolving the cause of her cancer. During the wrap-up of each session, I delivered suggestions that the IV treatment was working powerfully to strengthen her immune system while we continued to work together to clear out the remaining blocks to healing. That's what she wanted. That's what she expected. That's what she got. She is clear of the cancer now and has been for over a decade now. Was it the hypnosis or the IV treatments? I don't know. I don't care. Maybe it was both. She's healed. That's all that matters.

4. How is this problem impacting you in daily life?

When you're qualifying a client, this question serves to impress upon the client how important it is that they get the problem resolved. The more areas of life your client recognizes are being influenced by the problem, the more aware they become of how much of a problem it really is. This increases motivation for change.

Healing is about addressing the whole person, not merely the symptoms. As you resolve one piece of the problem, other problems will miraculously sort themselves out. This is because the one factor that all symptoms share is *the client*. But the client may not realize that they're connected until you point it out to them. Having a list of the areas being impacted by the problem tells you where to watch for change in the client's daily life. You can then use these things as evidence that change is happening and that the client is making progress. For example, you may be working on resolving the client's anger toward her boss but, because the issue is not yet completely resolved, her anger is still getting triggered by situations in daily life. Meanwhile, the client loses two dress sizes without dieting. True story. In this case, the anger toward the boss turned out to be unresolved anger toward her ex-husband, which tracked all the way back to her relationship with her mother in childhood. Surprise, surprise!

Find out what specific areas of the client's life are being affected as a result of having the problem. For example, how it impacting their work? Relationships? Sleep? Health? As you start resolving the client's presenting issue, change will occur, but it may not show up in the places you're expecting. This list will help you identify the benefits the client can expect as a result of making this change.

5. Do you have a spiritual practice?

Many clients will not volunteer information if they don't think it has anything to do with the problem. But research shows that having belief in a higher power can improve outcomes. My philosophy is that if the client has it, use it. Does the client have a spiritual practice of any kind? For example, meditation, yoga, church, prayer group, etc.

If the client considers themselves spiritual, what word do they use for their higher power? Some people strongly resist the "God word." There's always a reason for that. Sometimes it's because the client grew up in a religious household and, for some reason, it caused them pain. As a result, God means something different than safe, loving, and benevolent.

When I was teaching 7th Path Self-Hypnosis classes, I had a lot of clients tell me that the "charge" they had around the God word just dissolved away through the practice. If the client is more comfortable with some other word or phrase, that's okay. That's their word. If they have faith in "The Universe," use that. Some people like the word "Spirit." Some feel a connection to Jesus. It's not the word that's important. It's the meaning the client has given it.

I had a client suddenly realize that she needed to forgive God. She realized that she was blaming God for all the bad stuff that had happened in her life. This turned out to be a very interesting piece of the forgiveness work. It was also my first cancer client. The client was a healthcare worker and was undergoing chemotherapy and radiation treatments when she was seeing me. But she attributes her healing to the forgiveness work we did together.

Asking a person about their spiritual life can uncover meaningful information. For one client, this question opened the door to talking about childhood incest. For another, it conjured up happy memories of being in a Catholic school. Yet another reported how he was dragged off to church by a grandparent who turned out to be a key player at the root of the problem.

This question also acts as a natural segue into talking about the family system in childhood. Just ask, "What about growing up? Was your family religious in any way?" And now you've got them talking about childhood.

6. What was childhood like?

The Therapeutic Relationship establishes a safe place for the client's Inner Child to be heard, seen, and validated. This means that the Inner Child Work begins while you're conducting the intake. When you ask the client how they would describe childhood, you're inviting their Inner Child to be a part of the conversation. You'll get a variety of answers. Just know that everyone has unresolved stuff from childhood.

Every client needs to see you as stronger and wiser than they are. As a result, they will, to some degree, cast you in a parental role or "attachment figure." When that happens, the client's Inner Child will show itself. By modeling Healthy Parenting during the intake process, you can make it safe for the client to be real about how he feels. For example, I had a client tell me in a whiny tone, "I can't lose the weight because my wife does all the cooking." This is not a grownup speaking! This is the voice of a Child who feels powerless, unimportant, and subject to the control of others. (In this case, the root cause of the client's excess 100 pounds of weight was revealing itself as the unmet needs of an Inner Child.)

Don't Go There!

When a client tells you that they had a "perfect childhood," that their parents were loving and they never experienced any trauma or pain, that's a red flag. That's the Conscious Mind telling you, "Do not go there!" There's no need to challenge the client's perceptions. The Subconscious Mind knows the truth. It will show you during the regression. Just know to probe carefully. This is a tender area.

If the Conscious Mind believes that childhood was wonderful, okay. Just ask the client to tell you what their relationship with each parent was like growing up. Who do they talk about the most? Who they seem to avoid talking about or clearly *don't* want to talk about? This may be the person they have an issue with. For example, I had one client who did not want to talk about their father. She was adamant that she didn't need to talk about him. She'd been through therapy, forgiven him, the issue had been laid to rest, and was not up for discussion. But even mentioning dear old Dad clearly got her dander up. She got louder. Her face turned bright red. Her Subconscious Mind was straight-up telling me, "Don't go there!" Guess where the roots of her issue were? (Surprised the daylights out of her, too.)

No Recall

Sometimes the client doesn't remember much about childhood. It's possible that they had an uneventful childhood. More likely, there are traumatic experiences that happened so early in life that the client has no conscious recall of them. Trauma is an unavoidable fact of life growing up. It either builds resilience, or it knocks us down. Take birth, for example. Birth is inherently traumatic. Many lifelong problems can get seeded while you're trying to catch your first breath. Who remembers that?

Scientists have coined the phrase "childhood or infantile amnesia" to describe a veil of forgetfulness that descends around three. Anything before the age of three tends to be lost completely. Conscious recall of events from age three to around age seven tends to be spottier than they are later in life. The memories that are most likely to be preserved are highly emotional experiences.

Traumatic experiences are always emotionally charged events. Even when painful childhood experiences are remembered, the Adult Mind can judge these experiences as "no big deal." But it's the perceptions of the Child that so often generate problems for people later in life. This is because they form the basis of a person's Core Beliefs. Our Core Beliefs decide what we're going to get in life. They tell us who we need to be to get our needs met, what we deserve, and what to expect from others and life.

History of Abuse

Sometimes, it's clear that things were not so great in childhood and the client knows it. There was alcoholism. Abuse. Sibling rivalry. This is tough stuff for a kid to have to deal with alone. The isolation leaves deep wounds. I've had clients come to me to resolve childhood abuse issues. They were consciously aware of what had happened to them. They recognized that these past experiences were still impacting them and their ability to have loving relationships. They wanted to come to peace with their past. When a person has this level of willingness to face the past, you can move mountains, and you will transform lives for the better.

Family System

Some people will try to skip over childhood and talk about their relationship with a family member *now*. They'll talk about their relationship with Mom *now*, or their relationship with Dad *now*, or how great the relationship with their sister is *now*. That's another red flag. This tells you that the relationship has changed since childhood. You might have to probe a little to get to the truth but, if the client's description of childhood was less-than loving, their Inner Child might still be in distress. That may be at the root of the problem.

Work your way through the family system. Start with Mom and Dad. Then go through the list of siblings. What are their names? Are they alive or deceased? There may also be significant others who lived with the family of origin—for example, a grandparent, or a relative, or a boarder. Find out how they got along with these people. Siblings can be significant. For example, I've had clients who were bullied or abused by older siblings.

Some clients were born into large families and were neglected by their parents simply because there were just too many kids to care for. When you get a client from a large family, make a list of the siblings. Take note of the quality of each relationship. (I just put a plus or minus next to each name.) That way, you'll have something you can refer to when you're doing the regression work. Who's the oldest? Who's the youngest? Where is the client in the birth order? There's lots of research on the impact of birth order. Generally speaking, first-born children often take on the responsibility of being a parent to younger siblings. They take on the role of a babysitter or a surrogate mother. As a result, they feel they didn't get to have a childhood. The "baby" of the family is often special or privileged, making them a target for resentment. If the client was the result of an unplanned pregnancy, this could be interpreted as not being wanted.

Attachment Patterns

Research suggests that how a child is attached to his or her caregivers can have a major influence both during childhood and later in life. Insecure attachment can have a lasting effect on adult relationships later in life. For example, emotional problems like insecurity, self-doubt, anxiety, addiction, social impairment, and even disease can be rooted in early childhood attachment patterns.

Human beings need to attach or bond. Attachment patterns are learned responses based on the Child's experiences prior to twelve months of age. They reflect how the Child adapted to a specific relationship and are about that relationship, not the Child. The most important bond for a child is with the primary caregiver. Usually, that's Mother.

Attachment is not just about the connection between two people. It is a bond that involves the experience of distress when separated from that person. Infants and children stay close to their caregivers for protection. This increases their chances of survival. This emotional bond provides children with the safety they need to venture out and explore their environment. Clients who were adopted often have trauma related to being separated from Mom at birth. There's a bond between the child and mother that is established in the womb. Separation from Mom following birth is devastating for the Child.

Researchers have identified four different attachment styles which describe this emotional bond between children and their primary parent or caregiver. The following information can help you to identify the underlying, unmet needs of the client's Inner Child.

Secure Attachment

Ideal conditions result in Secure Attachment. This is where the Child feels safe in seeking connection with the attachment figure/Parent because the Parent is sensitive to and responds to the needs of the Child in a timely manner. This leads to healthy social, emotional, and cognitive development.

Avoidant Attachment

In Avoidant Attachment, the Child feels rejected or controlled by the parent. The problem is that the Parent isn't attuned to the needs of the Child. Either she doesn't seem to pick up on the Child's signals or fails to respond appropriately. Eventually, the Child stops trying to connect because it doesn't work out. The Child gives up and learns to tune out internally and externally.

This pattern results in socially controlling behavior, avoidance of others, not being very interactive, emotional distancing, and living in the head.

Ambivalent or Anxious Attachment

With this pattern, the Child amplifies internal and external cues, resulting in hyper-emotionality (the opposite of avoidant). In Ambivalent or Anxious Attachment, the parenting style is often so inconsistent that the Child cannot predict responses. This generates uncertainty and ambivalence toward the Parent. The Child then associates the anxiety with what's happening. For example, Mom's anger while feeding the baby gets anchored to food. Sometimes the Parent's emotional state intrudes on the Child's state. The Child then takes on the feelings of the Parent through emotional resonance.

This pattern often shows up in the teen years as insecurity, self-doubt, and inability to regulate emotions.

Disorganized Attachment

Disorganized Attachment indicates some kind of trauma. For example, physical, emotional, or verbal abuse; out-of-control behavior due to alcoholism; raging; violence, etc., which generated terror in the Child. The Child needs to attach because it cannot take care of itself. Because the Child is dependent on the Primary Caregiver for protection and soothing, it generates an internal conflict when the Parent is the source of threat.

This results in social, emotional, cognitive impairment. This pattern expresses as chaotic or confused behavior. The person can seem normal until triggered. For example, oscillating between clinginess and avoidance (move toward / run away).

7. *Significant Others?*

Relationship problems can be a reflection of insecure attachment in childhood. Partners can be chosen subconsciously to serve as Parental surrogates. The person then attempts to get their childhood needs met through their partner. This just never works because the problem has to do with the client's past.

The problem is rooted in the relationship to the primary caregiver in childhood, not the current relationship. If the client has been married several times, there may be a relationship pattern. How would the client describe their relationship with their spouse? How long have they been married? Are there any previous marriages? How many times have they been married?

Children

All sorts of unresolved stuff from past relationships can get carried over into present relationships, including the client's relationship with their children. Blended-family issues are always challenging. There can be conflicts over parenting style, which may have roots in the client's own childhood. Do they have children? How would the client describe their relationship with them? Have they ever lost a child?

If your client has ever had a miscarriage or an abortion, it could be a source of subconscious grief or guilt contributing to the client's symptoms.

8. *Are you using any medications?*

Many clients have been prescribed medication. Some will be taking multiple medications. If the client is taking multiple medications, make a list so that you can research what the drug is for and what the side effects may be. What are they, and what are they for? If the client doesn't know, find out. Some drugs need to be monitored by the client's prescribing physician. Some may cause you to think twice about working with the client at all.

All medications have side effects, and some may actually be contributing to the client's issue. For example, antidepressants or Selective Serotonin Reuptake Inhibitors (SSRIs) are the most commonly prescribed drug. Unfortunately, they work by putting a chemical lid on the client's ability to feel their emotions.

Antidepressants

Antidepressant medications work, but they do not discriminate. They work by putting a lid on *all* feelings, good and bad. The client doesn't feel bad anymore, but they don't feel good, either. They lose the ability to feel their good feelings. That's depressing. As a result, you'll get people coming to you because they're sick and tired of feeling like a zombie all the time. They want to get off the drugs so they can *feel* again. If you get a client who wants to get off antidepressants, make sure you have a doctor's referral. The client shouldn't just stop taking their medication. SSRIs have a half-life which means the client needs to be weaned off them gradually.

Antidepressants are not usually a problem when it comes to bringing up a feeling for regression work. The feelings are still there; they're just muted. I have had clients on multiple antidepressants who were able to find and feel enough emotional intensity to do the work.

Some clients just don't want to face their feelings. Intense feelings, especially those that are rooted in childhood trauma, can seem overwhelming because they were overwhelming for the client as a Child. The problem is that those unresolved emotions haven't gone anywhere. The internal pressure has been building up inside ever since. If the client is hesitant to allow feelings and emotions to come to awareness, educate them about how all feelings are good. Feelings and emotions are natural. They're meant to be helpful.

An emotion is a bio-chemical event that is felt in the body. It's a messenger signal coming from the brain, telling the body what to do. For example, hunger is a feeling that says you need to feed yourself. Fear is a feeling that says you need safety. Anger is a feeling that points to a need for healthy boundaries. Sadness is a feeling that points to a loss of connection. The signal tells the body how to respond so that you can take care of yourself.

Feelings are nature's biological feedback system. They're there for a reason. "Good" feelings tell us that we're satisfying our needs for safety, achievement, and connection. "Bad" feelings tell us we need to *do* something. We need to change something or take action in order to feel "good" again. When we ignore a feeling or try to avoid a feeling, the feeling doesn't go away. It just gets more insistent. It's like a Child tugging on the apron strings saying, "Mom. Mom. Mom. Mom." It's trying to get your attention so that you can meet an important need. That's good.

It's natural to feel our feelings. The feeling only becomes a problem when we resist it, or avoid it, or try to get rid of it. That's when it becomes insistent, like that kid going, "Mom. Mom. Mom. Mom." But like a Child, the feeling is never the problem. Feelings are normal and natural. All mammals experience them. It's only when you put a lid on your feelings that they become a problem. The way to put an end to an uncomfortable feeling is to feel it. Then, it's over.

The way to resolve an uncomfortable feeling is to simply face it and feel it. It's like a recurring nightmare. The "bad feeling" keeps chasing you, and you keep trying to get away from it, but you can't because it's not "out there." It's inside! The way to stop a nightmare is to turn around and face the feeling. Even the worst feeling won't last more than ninety seconds when you let yourself feel it. Simply feeling the truth of your feelings will put an end to the nightmares for good.

Recreational Substances

Before moving onto the next intake question, casually inquire about recreational substances such as drugs, alcohol, pharmaceuticals, or something else. You're not here to judge. You just want to know if the client is self-medicating in any way. If so, how? How frequently do they imbibe? Is it habitual or more social? Marijuana can cause paranoia in some people. It can make a person forgetful. It can also interfere with the hypnosis and mess with your results.

9. *What do you hope to accomplish as a result of us working together?"*

This is the turning point in the intake process. The client has shared his Pain Story with you. Talking about the pain of the problem has stirred up thoughts and feelings from the past. This can be an emotional experience for some of the clients. Now it's time to shift the energy so that you can end the intake process on a lighter note. Shift the focus onto the sense of possibility. The client may not know *how* it's possible, but you now have all the information you need to tell them. This is why the pre-talk comes after the intake process. Your intake allows you to customize the educational pre-talk to the specific needs and concerns of the client.

To wrap up the intake, invite the client's curiosity to be a part of the process by imagining what success might look like. That's what's motivating them to seek change. This gives you a positive note to end the intake on. When you ask the client to imagine, you're using the language of the Subconscious Mind. Interesting things can happen when you turn to the Subconscious Mind for help. How does the client want the Story to end? What will it look like once he's healed? How will he know when he has achieved his goal?

Ask the client, "If you could walk out of here today, completely transformed as a result of our work together, what would that look like?" Notice how we're coming full circle, back to the reason they came to see you in the first place? There's a feeling inside that's telling the client *it's possible*. It's possible to heal. It's possible to feel better. It's possible to get over this problem. That's all you need, that little bit of hope.

10. Anything else you think I should know?"

The intake process is a preliminary uncovering process that establishes a deeper level of intimacy between you and the client. As you move through the questions, the client will experience memories and emotions. As a result, insights can begin to bubble up to awareness. Other issues may be brought to light. But if the client doesn't mention it, you might miss something that could be critical to their healing. This is the client's opportunity to come clean with you.

Some clients just need more time to open up fully. The final question invites the client to share freely. Most of the time, the client will say, "No, I think we've covered everything . . ." Sometimes they'll say, "Gosh, I didn't realize how much those things still bother me!" And every once in a while, the client will say, "Well . . . actually . . . there *is* something else . . . ." Sometimes the answer to this question can point to the *real* problem! For example, a client who presented with a pattern of leaving relationships said tearfully, "I have never been able to feel close to my mom." Boom. Guess who was at the center of the client's emotional storm?

Summary

Healing is about addressing the whole person, not merely treating a symptom. Your intake process is a strategy for establishing a deeper level of intimacy with both the Conscious and Subconscious minds. Listening to the client's Pain Story helps to satisfy the Conscious Mind's need for control to ensure it won't try to run the show. It also allows the Subconscious Mind to learn that you can be trusted to guide the client safely. This is the basis of the Therapeutic Relationship.

As the client is sharing their Pain Story, feelings and memories are naturally going to bubble up to conscious awareness from the Subconscious level of Mind. These emotional memories have everything to do with the client's presenting issue and help you to guide the healing process confidently and effectively.

The intake is much more than taking a history of the client's problem. This is a preliminary uncovering procedure that allows you to identify the Symptom Resolution Keys. For example:

- How is the problem expressing as a Symptom Pattern?
- When did symptoms first appear and how?
- What methods have worked in the past?
- What methods do you need to avoid?
- Where can you look for signs of change?
- What is the client's source of power for change?
- What was the client's family system like growing up?
- What's going on in the client's family system now?
- What emotions are connected to the client's presenting issue?
- Are there any known incidents of trauma?
- Is the client self-medicating in any way?
- What outcome holds hope for the client?
- What hasn't the client mentioned?

CHAPTER 7:
Set Up to Wrap Up

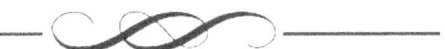

Once you have completed the process of guiding the client through the intake questions, you'll have the information you need to guide the healing process effectively. But before you start guiding the client into hypnosis, take a few minutes to identify the critical information that will support you in guiding the healing process effectively.

Set up to wrap up your sessions powerfully by creating a Session Worksheet. This only takes a few minutes to conduct. Your Session Worksheet supports you in getting a lasting result by organizing the information you need in every session onto a single sheet of paper. This puts the information you need to guide the healing session effectively at your fingertips. And you can use it to wrap up your sessions powerfully – without ever needing a script.

Scripts are a great way to learn how to deliver suggestions effectively. They're a great place to look for ideas and can teach you how to craft an elegant suggestion. But you don't need them because the client will give you everything you need. During the intake process, you will gather the three critical pieces of information you need to wrap up every session in a way that is relevant to the client's desired outcome.

These three critical pieces of information remind the client of why they are taking this journey with you. They are the client's:

1. Therapeutic goal.
2. Conditions for change.
3. Benefits of change.

Where are you going? What is it that the client wants to accomplish by doing this work with you? This is the client's Therapeutic Goal.

What needs to happen in order to achieve this goal? How are they going to achieve their objective? What actions or behaviors are going to contribute to creating this change? These are the client's Conditions for Change.

How will you know when you get there? What rewards does the client hope to enjoy as a result of having made this change? What's the motivating factor? These are the client's Benefits of Change.

Once you have gathered this information, you'll have everything you need to wrap up each session in a way that speaks to the client's most important needs, wants, and desires.

Therapeutic Goal

A mistake that too many hypnotherapists make is failing to establish a clearly defined Therapeutic Goal. If you've ever felt like you were spinning your wheels, trying to get a result, it's probably because you weren't specific enough. It's the leading cause of frustration and failure for both therapists and clients.

You and the client are about to embark on an amazing journey of self-discovery and self-healing. Where are you going? If you don't know where you're going, how will you get there? You need to have a clearly defined, specific goal to focus on before you go to work on the client's issue. Before you enter into the territory of the Subconscious Mind, get clear. What's the client's desired outcome? What's the destination? What does the client want to accomplish by doing this work with you?

As you navigate through the healing process, the client's Therapeutic Goal will act as your north star, keeping you pointed in the right direction.

Once you have completed the intake process, return to the client's issue. Come full circle, back to the problem. That's what brought the client to you in the first place. Ask the client to make a statement, in their own words, to define what their specific Therapeutic Goal is. What's their desired outcome? Make sure that it's specific. Generalizations won't get you where you want to go. The more specific you can be, the more effective you'll be because everything you do in the healing process will be pointing toward this one thing. To establish a clearly defined Therapeutic Goal, the client needs to pick one specific goal to focus on. But what if the client has more than one issue?

Multiple Issues

When a client is wrestling with multiple issues, they may have difficulty coming up with a clearly defined Therapeutic Goal. All of these issues need to be recognized as valid concerns. But trying to deal with more than one issue at a time makes it very difficult to get any traction. If you want to make progress, you need to focus on one goal at a time. You can help the client to set aside all other concerns by making a list of all their issues.

Making a list is a way of honoring those problems. You're giving them a place to go by writing them down. Validating each issue of concern makes it easier for the client to let it go so that you can focus on one specific Therapeutic Goal. Writing the client's problems down doesn't get rid of them. It just gives them a place to go. The client is handing them over to you for safekeeping. Just listing all their issues, worries, and concerns can help the client to sort through their thoughts and come to clarity.

Once you have created a list, you need to do something with it. The next step is to go through the list and ask the client to prioritize each of their issues. Which issue is the worst? Which issue is the oldest? The process of prioritizing each issue of concern can help to identify where to begin the healing process. One of the ways you can do this is to use a Subjective Unit of Distress (SUD). Ask the client to rate each problem on a scale of one to ten. For example, "On a scale of one to ten, how much of a problem is this?" Which of the complaints is the most pressing? Which one is wreaking the most havoc in their life? That might be the place to begin the healing process.

The problem that will get the client the most bang for their therapeutic buck will be the big, painful emotional problem. Any issue with a big emotional charge can yield a dramatic shift because that's where the energy is trapped. There's more pressure looking for a way out. But if it's something really big, there's going to be more resistance to facing it. Sometimes, it's more effective to start with something smaller. This gives you something to build on by allowing the client to experience some success before addressing the hairier issue.

Once your client has experienced some success with you, you'll find that other issues will be much easier to deal with. The client's faith in the process will be based on first-hand experience, instilling more confidence. They'll have developed skills working with you as a team, making your job easier. You will have drained off some of the accumulated internal stress and pressure they've been carrying around inside, making other issues easier to resolve.

Nothing builds success like success, and nothing instills confidence better than proof. A small win can pave the way for bigger wins. It all depends on the client. If you need to increase the client's trust or confidence, a smaller issue will allow you to experience a quicker result. If the client is having an emotional catharsis during the intake process, that's where their Subconscious Mind wants to go. It's telling you, loud and clear, "Here's the problem!" If the Subconscious Mind is pushing feelings and emotions up to the surface of awareness, it's because it wants you to take care of it. Use it!

Creating a Laundry List can help you to identify the client's Therapeutic Goal. Everything you do is then directed toward one specific goal allowing you to get a more rapid result. Once you have resolved this issue, you can come back to the client's Laundry List to see what, if anything, is still left. The client can then decide whether or not they want or need to work on another issue.

The Laundry List Technique

1. **Make a list.** List all the problems that the client is struggling with. Give them a place to go.
2. **Prioritize.** Ask the client to put their problems in order of priority. Take a SUD. On a scale of one to ten, how bad is it?
3. **Pick one.** Depending on the client, choose a specific issue to start with. The one with the biggest emotional charge will yield a more dramatic result. Focusing on a smaller issue can help to instill confidence by allowing the client to experience a quicker win.
4. **Make a statement.** Ask the client to give you a clear statement of intent. Words have power. In their own words, what do they want as a result?

Everything on the client's Laundry List has one thing in common—the client. This means that some of those issues of concern are going to be connected. There will be a central theme holding them all together. Because the Subconscious Mind tends to generalize change, when you resolve a Subconscious pattern or theme, it has a ripple effect throughout the Mind-Body system. When this happens, other issues can start to fall away. This means that, as you focus on resolving one specific issue, other issues will start to shift. Some will just resolve on their own.

The client's Laundry List also tells you where to look for signs of change. You need to watch for them, though, because the client may not realize that these changes result from the work you are doing together. The client may not realize it, but *they* are changing. Why else would it be that these other problems are falling away? What you're doing is working!

During your Session Wrap Up, help the client connect the dots. Celebrate every change for the better, no matter how small! Treat it like the client just won an Olympic Gold medal! Help the client to recognize that their own Mind is creating these changes. Even a small change can be a big win that will contribute to the client's overall happiness in life. Help the client to realize that this is the power of their own Mind. The rewards of change are far greater than they might have imagined! If the client has been struggling with a complex issue, this can be just the encouragement they need to see it through and achieve the results. They may still have symptoms associated with the presenting problem, but something has changed at a Subconscious level of Mind. *They* are changing. Use this as exciting evidence that progress is being made! This can encourage the client to hang in there long enough to achieve their Therapeutic Goal.

Once you have identified the client's Therapeutic Goal, formulate a goal statement for your Session Worksheet by asking the client, "In a nutshell, what do you want?" Then test it with a Subjective Unit of Truth (SUT). Ask your client, "On a scale of one to ten, where ten is "absolute conviction," how *true* does this goal statement feel?"

Conditions for Change

The client's Therapeutic Goal tells you what the client wants to accomplish. It defines where you are going. The Conditions for Change List defines how you are going to get there. What needs to change for the client to realize their Therapeutic Goal?

The Conditions for Change is a list of changes that the client recognizes will help them to achieve their goal. You can use this information to plot a course toward their final destination. The Conditions for Change are specifically tied to the client's Therapeutic Goal. Ask the client, "What would have to be true for your Therapeutic Goal to happen?"

Create a list of specific actions or behaviors that the client believes are necessary for her to achieve her goal. What behaviors or actions does the client believe will contribute to her success?

- What needs to change?
- What does the client need to be doing?
- What are they already doing that they need to do more of?

- What do they need to stop doing?
- What could they do, instead?

This gives you a list of strategies that the client is already invested in. The client's belief gives them power.

The purpose of defining the Conditions for Change is to make the client responsible for making the change. This is laying the foundation for the Therapeutic Contract. The client usually knows what needs to change for them to achieve their goal. While you can make it easier for the client to take action, you can't do it for them. For example, if you're working on a behavioral issue like weight loss, the client already knows what she *should* be doing. She just hasn't been able to do it. That's why she needs your help. In this case, the client knows that she needs to change her lifestyle habits. She knows where the trouble spots are and where she is likely to get sabotaged.

The Conditions for Change list gives you the information you need to formulate post-hypnotic suggestions, homework assignments and test the results between sessions. What behaviors contribute to the problem? What newer, healthier behaviors will contribute to successfully achieving the Therapeutic Goal? What has she done in the past that worked? What does the client need to be doing, from now on, that she's not doing now? What needs to happen for the client to heal? Who does she need to become to have the change she desires?

Not every issue requires behavioral change, but the Conditions for Change List can also give you a way to test the client's expectations and uncover any hidden issues. For example, if the client is expecting you to do all the work, that's a problem. If they think you're going to wave your magic wand and *make* them change, you need to resolve that. If the client expects to keep eating two large pizzas and a gallon of ice cream, every night, that's unreasonable. You can't override the laws of nature. Conditions for Change must be realistic.

An unrealistic expectation to watch for is the requirement that someone *else* change before the client can be happy. This is a subtle block that can prevent the client from being successful. For example, I had a weight loss client who was married to an alcoholic. She was adamant that she would not lose the weight until her husband stopped drinking. That's an unrealistic expectation. If the client's ability to have what she wants is dependent on someone else changing, guess who has all the power? This also points to a grievance. The person that the client held responsible for the problem was someone who needed to be forgiven before the client could take back control of her life. This client believed that she was fat because her husband was an alcoholic. It was his fault. By abdicating self-responsibility, she was keeping herself stuck in victim mode.

In order to get free of the problem, the client needed to take back her power. To do that, she needed to let go of the grievance and let hubby be however he chose to be. That's realistic. Hold your clients accountable for creating change. What this client needed to hear was, "He isn't in the chair. If he needs to change, he'll have to book his own appointment. The only person that can change right now is YOU. You're the one with the problem. You're the one in the chair. The choice is yours." She got it.

The client's Conditions for Change list can give you guidelines for creating positive change. Are the client's expectations realistic? What needs to happen for the client to realize their goal? You can use this information to formulate suggestions, establish milestones of change and test the results.

Formulate Suggestions

Your client provides the script. Suggestions that come from the client are always more acceptable than anything you might think up! Just ask – "What needs to change?" What does the client need to stop doing or start doing to be successful?

Make a list. What new behaviors will contribute to achieving their goal? For example, a weight-loss client might tell you that he needs to stop having three helpings at dinner or that taking the dog for a walk before dinner would help him to relax, putting him more in control over his eating choices. Then ask yourself, *Is the behavior doable?*

Is the client capable of making this change? Is there anything that might prevent him from doing so? Is he willing to take action? If so, you have everything you need to formulate suggestions specific to that client's needs.

Establish Milestones of Change

Some Conditions for Change will be small, easy changes to install. Others will be more challenging and take longer to implement. A small win, early on, can increase client motivation and pave the way for greater successes. Giving the client a taste of success can give them the boost that they need to tackle more difficult challenges. If you start with something small, you'll find that it easier to get the bigger wins. For example, a weight-loss client with over 100 pounds to lose has a more challenging issue. It's going to take some time for the client to safely release the weight.

In this case, you can chunk down into smaller, easier-to-achieve milestones. Think increments of change. A shorter-term goal of, say, the first twenty pounds establishes a milestone that gets the client moving in the right direction. Some weight-loss programs call this a "quick-start." They take advantage of the higher motivation at the beginning of a program to get some quick wins for the client. Successfully achieving one milestone gives the client permission to allow more change. Conditions for Change act as positive actions that you can line up as milestones toward the client's larger goal.

Short-Term Coping Strategies

The client's Conditions for Change can also be used to formulate short-term coping strategies for dealing with situational stress. While you can't change outer conditions with hypnosis, you can certainly help the client cope with a toxic environment by changing their internal responses to triggers in daily life. For example, the weight-loss client mentioned earlier was on a mission to make her alcoholic husband change. It wasn't what the client was eating that was the problem. It was what was eating her. As a result, she and hubby were constantly getting into fights. The client was picking fights in an attempt to get her needs met. These needs had roots in childhood, but her frustration and anger, as an adult, generated anxiety which was driving her to self-medicate with food. In this case, the Condition for Change was to change her response to her husband's behavior. This gave us a milestone to work towards as we journeyed toward her Therapeutic Goal. It also provided a way to test the results.

Test the Results

As we released the internal anger and anxiety, the client felt calmer and more in control. The need to struggle to get her needs met started to melt away. As a result, the fighting with hubby stopped. This turned the tables on her relationship. As long as she was out of control and picking fights, her husband was able to dismiss her as irrational. When she stopped demanding that he change to make her happy, she started to find other ways to satisfy her own needs. That's when her husband started trying to sabotage things in an attempt to reinstall the old pattern. This was useful feedback because it allowed us to identify where her specific triggers were. These were then used to guide the process so we could get to the underlying issue, which, of course, had nothing to do with hubby.

I had a weight client who needed to stop eating candy. Every night, she sat in front of the TV and ate candy. She knew she needed to stop this behavior. She just couldn't do it. You can't just suggest that away. Trying to suggest away an emotion won't get you long-term results. If anything, it will just increase the internal resistance. And this client was not going to accept a suggestion to just stop eating candy.

She had already been through Cognitive Behavioral Therapy and counseling. The very thought of giving up the candy increased the anxiety. The reason behavioral approaches failed was because the problem wasn't the behavior. The behavior was a Subconscious Solution to the real problem. That's what was driving her to turn to candy for solace. Sugar calms anxiety.

The anxiety wasn't the problem, either. The problem was what was behind the anxiety, which was a load of accumulated, unresolved fear and anger looking for a way out. While her Condition for Change was to stop eating the candy every night, it took on a different function.

Instead of trying to install it as a new behavior, which the client was highly resistant to, we used it as a way to test the results. This gave us a way to measure the client's progress. The client knew that when the real problem was truly resolved, she'd find it easy to do what, consciously, she wanted to do – stop binging on sweets. The behavior would fall away on its own. And it did.

The day she was able to put the candy bars into a garbage bin, and take it to the curb, was the day that she knew the problem was gone for good. A year later, she was fifty pounds lighter, physically and emotionally.

Benefits of Change

The client's Therapeutic Goal tells you what they want. Their Conditions for Change tell you what needs to happen so that they can have it. The client's Benefits List provides you with the motivating factors. Each benefit acts as a reminder of why the client is taking this journey with you. These are all the real reasons the client is taking this journey with you. What does their "happily ever after" look like? Why it's worth it to do the work necessary to make this change? Human beings are motivated to seek pleasure and avoid pain. What are the rewards of change? Create a list.

- What are the benefits of achieving the Therapeutic Goal?
- How is life going to improve as a result of realizing this goal?
- How will the client know when they have arrived at their destination?

For example, how will they feel when they look in the mirror and realize they have made this change? What will other people think? How will they respond differently in certain situations in life?

Be Specific

These are the pictures and imaginings of who the client becomes as a result of having made those changes for themselves. This means they need to be specific. "I'll be happy" just isn't specific enough to motivate a person to create change. What does "happy" *look* like? How will they know when they *have* it? Think in terms of health, relationship, sleep, mood, and so on.

Ask your client, "How will their life improve?" For example, work, health, sleep, mood, relationships, etc. The more benefits the client can come up with, the more leverage you will have. The greater their motivation to change, the more hopeful they will feel. Create a list of at least seven benefits.

The Benefits of Change need to be personally and emotionally motivating. They're for the client. Not their spouse, children, parents, doctor, or anyone else. They should feel really good. Exciting. Empowering. What will they be doing/having/being as a result of having made this change? These are all the reasons for taking action and allowing change to happen.

Go for Willpower

Sometimes, the client will try to give you a list of all the things they won't have to put up with anymore. They'll say, "I won't have to do this anymore." Or, "I won't have to deal with that anymore." Or, "I won't feel so bad all the time." "Won't power" won't get them what they want. What you're looking for a list of specific positive benefits.

When a client gives you a "won't" list, realize that they've been stuck for too long. They're in the habit of focusing on what they don't want or have. The problem with this habituated point of view is that it's self-reinforcing. The more they focus on what they don't want, the more they reinforce that truth in their own Mind, so don't slide on this! Hold the client responsible for coming up with real motivators. These are the rewards of change that get the client inspired and moving in the direction of their heart's desire. That's willpower.

Get a Felt-Sense

The rewards of change are always emotional. When the client imagines the benefits of having achieved their Therapeutic Goal, it should have a positive emotional charge to it. It should excite the client because the rewards of change are not external; they're internal. They should conjure images of better times to come. They should feel hopeful. Once you have completed the Benefits List, test each one by reviewing the list with the client to get a felt sense of each benefit.

Instruct your client to close their eyes and listen as you read each of their benefits out to them. Tell them to, "Just listen and notice how each one feels." Remind the client that you don't want them to think; you want them to notice how each benefit feels as they picture it in their Mind. Each picture should have a little "spike" of excitement to it. If it doesn't, it's not sufficiently motivating. Get more specific and increase the client's willpower.

As you read through the list, the Subconscious Mind will often begin to identify more benefits that you can add to the client's list of Benefits of Change. The more, the merrier!

The Big Bang Benefit

Once you have reviewed their Benefits list, ask the client, "Which of these benefits feels most important?" Which one has the most juice? If the client isn't sure, repeat the reviewing process. Instruct the client to close their eyes and go inside, as you read out each benefit, once more, only *this time* you want them to feel the answer to this question, "Which one feels like it's the most important one?" Which of these important, personal benefits generates the biggest spike of emotion as they picture themselves doing, having, or being? That's their Big Bang Benefit! If the client isn't sure, you can take a Subjective Unit of Pleasure (SUP). On a scale of one to ten, where ten is total bliss, how pleasurable is that benefit?

Summary

Before you begin the healing process, you need a clearly defined specific goal to guide the healing process. What does the client want as a result of doing this work with you? This establishes the Therapeutic Goal.

If a client has more than one issue, create a Laundry List. Then, focus on one at a time. If you try to work on more than one issue at a time, you'll just end up spinning your wheels. There is an easier way.

Big emotional issues will yield a more dramatic result but, sometimes, choosing a smaller issue to work on is more effective. Establishing a foundation of success gives you something to build on. Remember, nothing builds success like success.

As a common thread will connect some issues on the list, resolving one issue can neutralize several others at the same time, making your job easier! If you're dealing with an issue that has a lot of moving parts, it can keep the client in the game long enough to successfully resolve the whole pattern.

Once you have formulated the client's Therapeutic Goal, take a SUT. How true does their goal statement feel?

The Conditions for Change are specifically tied to the client's Therapeutic Goal. Ask the client, "What would have to be true for your Therapeutic Goal to happen?" This gives you a list of changes that the client is already invested in. You can use the client's Conditions for Change list to:

- Uncover unrealistic expectations.
- Identify secondary gain issues.
- Formulate suggestions.
- Establish milestones of achievement.
- Formulate short-term coping strategies.
- Increase motivation.
- Test the results.
- Provide proof of change.

The client's Benefits of Change List defines the motivating factors driving the Therapeutic Goal. How will the client's life improve? What areas will be impacted positively by these changes?

Create a list of at least seven benefits. These are the rewards the client gets to enjoy for having taken this journey with you.

Benefits must be specific. They should conjure a picture of doing, having, or being.

Benefits are personal rewards. They're not for anyone else and they should feel really good, exciting, empowering.

The benefits are positive and inspiring. Focus on "I will" rather than "I won't."

The rewards of change are emotional. When the client imagines their benefit, they should feel excited.

Once you have completed the client's Benefit List, review the list one last time to identify the most important benefit. Look for the spike of emotion. That's the Big Bang Benefit. If the client isn't sure, take a SUP! Which benefit promises the greatest amount of pleasure?

Forgiveness means being okay with it – all of it. Ultimately, it's about respecting yourself. When you deeply and completely love and accept yourself, you don't let other people walk all over you or treat you like dirt. You can demand respect. If they refuse, they can go to hell without you choosing to join them. – **The Devil's Therapy**

CHAPTER 8:
Set Up for Forgiveness Work

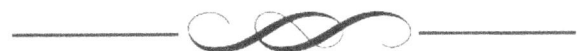

There are people in the client's life who may be contributing to the problem. These people will show up during regression sessions but, often, they will be revealed during the intake process. You can transfer this information onto the back of your Session Worksheet for easy reference during your sessions. To save time, you can even do this while you're conducting the intake.

Your Session Worksheet also gives you a place to keep track of any Forgiveness Work that's been done. Keeping a list of key players on your Session Worksheet means that, should the client go back into an event involving this person, you won't have to remember who they are. You can see at a glance whether this person has angel or demon status in the client's life.

Key Players

Key Players are important relationships contributing to the client's Pain Story. These will include Mom, Dad, siblings, and any significant others such as grandparents, spouse, ex-spouses, etc. What are their first names? Are they living or dead? If alive, what is the client's relationship with them now? If deceased, when did they die? The loss of a parent can trigger unresolved childhood issues. For example, the subconscious realization that Mom will never meet the client's childhood needs.

Unresolved grief could be contributing to the client's presenting issue. For example, I had a client who was the last living member of her family. One by one, each had succumbed to disease over a period of fifteen years. That's a lot of accumulated loss to have to deal with!

Quality of Relationship

Make a note of the quality of each relationship by using a plus or a minus sign next to each name. For example, if the client's relationship with that person was positive, put a plus sign next to their name (+). This person would then represent an internal resource available to the client.

If the relationship is conflicted in some way, put a plus and a minus sign next to their name (+/-). For example, the client may realize that they love a parent, but they don't get along with them for some reason. It may be that the relationship has changed. Maybe they had a problem in childhood, but they've since resolved their differences. Make a note of this as there may still be a conflict at the Subconscious level of Mind.

If there is a person who hurt the client in some way, put a double negative next to their name (-/-). For example, clients will tell you a parent or a sibling abused them. Often, they're still carrying the pain of those experiences.

Other Players

The back of the worksheet is a place to keep any information that is relevant to the client's healing process. You can continue to add more information as it arises through the regression work. For example, other Players or sources of support might be revealed through the process.

Forgiveness

The Session Worksheet also gives you a place to keep track of any forgiveness work done. You can then test the results to ensure a lasting result.

Insights & Evidence

The client may have insights that you can reinforce as additional resources. When a client experiences an insight, something has changed internally. Make a note of it. When a client realizes positive change has occurred between sessions, add it to the back of your Session Worksheet. You can then use these realizations and recognitions to formulate suggestions during your Session Wrap Up. Reminding the client that change is occurring and that they are moving in the right direction can help increase motivation while reinforcing the changes that are occurring.

Summary

The back of your Session Worksheet gives you a place to keep track of additional information that can support you in guiding the healing process. For example:

- Key Players growing up.
- Quality of each relationship.
- Other Players revealed through the regression work.
- People who need to be forgiven.
- People who have been forgiven.
- Positive resources and sources of support.
- Insights and evidence of change.
- Between session tests.

This additional information can be used to formulate suggestions during your Session Wrap Up.

"You can't make a person heal. Nobody can. The power to heal is in the Mind of the client. To heal, the client must be willing to allow healing to happen. That can take time. While healing can happen in an instant. Most of the time, what's required is a process of accruing enough 'sweepings' to shift the balance. For this reason, The Devil's Therapy is not a quick-fix solution; it's a client-centered solution." ~ **The Devil's Therapy**

CHAPTER 9:
Ditch the Script

You're ready to ditch the script and start offering targeted suggestions that are relevant to the client's healing. Once you have completed your Session Worksheet, have everything you need during a session right at your fingertips! You are set up to wrap up your session powerfully without ever needing a script. Not only will this make your job easier, but the suggestions you deliver will also pack a real punch because they come from the client. They're not coming out of some generic script. They're specifically what your client knows and wants.

When you use your Session Worksheet to create suggestions, you'll be speaking to the client's hopes and dreams. You'll be conjuring up pictures of what it looks like to have achieved what they want and what it feels like to have succeeded. Your Session Worksheet holds all the information you need to craft suggestions that are specific to the client's Therapeutic Goal, Conditions for Change, Benefits of Change, Forgiveness Work, available resources, evidence of change, and more.

The Icing on the Cake

Your Session Wrap Up is a process of putting the icing on the cake. It occurs just before you emerge the client from hypnosis. This is where you do a brief review to make whatever happened in the session relevant to the client's issue and set up for the next session.

Therapeutic Goal

Begin by reminding the client of why they are taking this journey with you. This is the client's Therapeutic Goal. It's where they want to get to, where you're leading them. The client's willingness to do the work necessary to achieve their goal is based on their Therapeutic Goal. Make whatever happened in the session relevant by offering the suggestion that the Subconscious Mind now has the information it needs to begin making the desired changes. Review any shifts, insights, or better feelings that occurred during the session and use it as evidence that change is already occurring. Then encourage a deeper level of healing by instructing the Subconscious Mind to take all these changes and integrate them in a way that is most beneficial to the client—physically, mentally, emotionally, and spiritually.

Remind the client that all that is needed is to decide on the direction, then commit to taking the next step. Then suggest that, as they have already taken the first step, the journey has already begun. Many things have happened. Many things are about to occur. Encourage the client to feel confident that change is already occurring and that success is only a matter of time. Then, instruct the Subconscious Mind to continue the healing between sessions.

A Journey of a Thousand Miles Begins with a Single Step – **Chinese Proverb**

Benefits of Change

The Therapeutic Goal is not merely a change the client wants to make. It's their vision for themselves of the future. It's a picture of the person they will become as a result of having made this change.

The Benefits List tells you why the client wants to realize this dream and gives you all the reasons for doing the work necessary to create change. This is what will keep the client committed to achieving their goal.

Imagination and emotion are the languages of the Subconscious Mind. The rewards of change are always emotional because emotion is the motivating factor of the Subconscious Mind. The Benefits of Change, when imagined, should generate pleasurable feelings and emotions. They should feel exciting. Invite the client to vividly imagine what it will be like to have achieved their goal. Instruct the client to bring in all of their five senses—seeing, hearing, tasting, smelling, feeling—and experience it *as if* it were already true. Then, go through their list of benefits and invite the client to experience what it's like to be enjoying the rewards of having achieved their goal.

What the mind expects to happen tends to be realized. — **Gerald Kein**

This can be an interactive process, or you can just deliver a few suggestions. It depends on how much time you have left in the session. The objective is to end the session on a high note. At the very least, you want to emerge the client from a session feeling hopeful. What feelings are associated with the picture they're holding in their mind? What emotions correspond to the experience of having made that change? Amplify those good feelings!

Social approval is another strong motivator. Invite the client to imagine sharing this change with loved ones. Give them the experience of what it's like to have others recognizing and approving of their having made these changes. Help the client discover how this reinforces the pride of accomplishment that they *already* feel for having given themselves this wonderful gift.

Conditions for Change

The Conditions for Change list tells you how the client is going to get where they're going. This gives you a way to strategize for success by setting up milestones of achievement and testing the results. You don't have to make the client do anything to change. You just need to create space for a new sense of possibility, then fill that space with positive suggestions. Think of this as filling the client's tank. Fill it with their permission to allow change to happen. Fill it permission to courageously take those first few steps or enthusiastically take action to make those changes. That's what will allow them to have all the rewards they want!

When the client imagines having the results, they experience a reward state. This reduces resistance to taking action to create those changes. How did they realize this change for themselves? How proud do they feel for having made this change? How much better is life for them now? What other rewards are they now enjoying? How is achieving their Goal, and all the benefits, a natural consequence of having made the right choices? The healthier choices?

See what I mean? You won't find this in any generic script. This stuff is gold because you get it from the client. That's where the answers lie. All you have to do is help the client connect all the dots and their Subconscious Mind will do the rest. As you resolve the internal blocks that have been preventing them from achieving their goal, the positive images that come to mind will become more believable to the client. As the resistance to allowing change dissolves away, the behaviors that contributed to the problem will fall away. The newer, healthier behaviors that will contribute to the client's desired outcome will then become more doable in daily life.

Connect the Dots

Connecting the Dots is a type of puzzle where a line is drawn to connect two dots. As more dots are connected by lines, the shape of an object is revealed. This is what your Session Wrap Up should do. You're connecting whatever happened in the client's session to their Therapeutic Goal, Conditions for Change, and Benefits of Change to create a picture of the future the client is living in. You can use the following 3 Rs in the Wrap Up Review to set your clients up to realize a much brighter future.

The 3 Rs in the Wrap Up Review

The Wrap-Up Review gives you a way to help the client to connect all the dots by reviewing whatever happened during the session. You can then turn it into a learning experience to empower the client.

The first R in Review is Relevant.

Whatever the client discovers during a session has everything to do with the reason they're seeing you. That's their Therapeutic Goal. The objective is to take what was revealed during the session and make it relevant to the client's issue. Use your Session Wrap Up to help the client connect the dots between what happened during the session and their waking life. You can then use the client's own realizations as evidence of their ability to create the kind of change they want.

A script won't do this because it's just your word. But if the client makes these connections for themselves, then it must be true. Be creative with your Session Wrap Up and use whatever came up in the client's session to guide them in the direction of their Therapeutic Goal. If the client regressed to a painful event from the past, you could use it as exciting evidence that their Subconscious Mind wants the problem resolved. Use it as evidence that the client has given themselves permission to heal the *real* problem and set themselves free of the past.

Whatever the client discovered during the session is meant to be helpful. It's pointing them in the direction of their Therapeutic Goal. If something painful was revealed, suggest that it has everything to do with the problem the client has been struggling with. Help the client to realize that it's not their fault. It's because something happened, or they were just a kid, or they were too young.

First, connect the session to the client's Therapeutic Goal. Whatever has just occurred in the session is going to make it easier for them to achieve their goal. Things have been brought to light. Shifts have occurred. Something has happened. Tie it to their goal. For example: Why are they taking this journey with you? How will taking back a part of their life that's been missing or out of control help the client to achieve their Therapeutic Goal?

Second, connect the session to the client's Conditions for Change. What actions are going to contribute to them achieving their goal? For example: Why do they find it so much easier to take action because of what happened in the session? Are they more relaxed? More self-aware? More motivated? How are they changing? Do they feel proud for taking action to achieve their Therapeutic Goal? What else is changing because of these things?

Third, connect the session to the client's Benefits of Change. How is making this change going to reward them? For example: What are the benefits of making this change? Why do they feel so much better about themselves? How are their relationships changing for the better? How much healthier do they feel? Where are they discovering sources of empowerment in daily life to support them? What's their most important benefit? Who are they becoming as a result of taking this journey with you?

The second R in Review is Revelation.

A revelation is a surprising, unknown fact. Think of this as "the aha!" What did the client discover? What did they learn? What do they know now that they didn't know before? How are they changing for the better? What else might be changing as a result? Whatever the client discovered during the session is new information that's just been revealed to them by their Subconscious Mind. This forms the basis for suggestions that begin with, "Now you know . . ."

At the end of each session, go through your notes and gather up any insights, learnings, or realizations that were brought to light during the session, and transform them into revelations by reminding the client, "Now you know . . ."

> For example, "**Now you know** . . . you have this wonderful ability. You can use it to create the kind of change you want."

"**Now you know** . . . those things that happened when you were two years old were not your fault. You were just a Child, then. But you're not a Child anymore. You're an adult, able to make better choices for yourself and your well-being from now on. (Tie to Conditions for Change list)."

"**Now you know** . . . you're allowed to feel your feelings. You're allowed to heal. Those feelings that got trapped inside have everything to do with (the problem). You're changing now. Give yourself permission to finally become the person you were always meant to be by releasing everything that has been getting in the way of you feeling good about you (tie to Conditions for Change list)."

"I want you to realize what a wonderful gift you have given yourself today. You gave yourself permission to feel better today. You'll continue to enjoy all the benefits of having created this change because **now you know** . . . you have discovered within you this wonderful ability. You can use it to create the kind of change you want. This allows you to begin to feel healthier, happier, and more successful in every way. And as we continue to work together, releasing all remaining blocks, more and more, you can discover what it's like to really be enjoying life free of the past."

"Take a moment, now, to imagine what it's like to be moving forward with your life—moving into your future, taking with you all these wonderful, positive changes that you have created for yourself. And as you do, experience what it's like to be doing things free of the past. Let yourself experience it vividly, using all your senses as if it's already true. Sense it, see it, hear it, feel it. Use all your senses. And experience what it's like to be enjoying all the benefits (go through Benefits List)."

"That's good. The Subconscious Mind now has the information it needs(pause). Just take a few moments to just be in that place, and relax, and notice how much better you feel. Feel good?"

When a client regresses into a painful past event, you might not have enough time to process everything. If you need to wrap up a session before everything has been cleared, that's okay. Just use what was revealed to instill confidence in the process. For example, you can reframe any painful event as a breakthrough moment in the client's healing. Their Subconscious Mind has just revealed something that has everything to do with their Therapeutic Goal! What have they just discovered? What are they learning? This is exciting evidence that change is occurring.

No matter what is brought to light during a session, the goal is to tie everything together in a way that makes it relevant to the client's healing goal. Connect all the dots by using the suggestion, "Now you know . . ." Validate any insights the client might have had. Turn them into revelations. This empowers the client.

The third R in Review is Reinforce.

To get a rapid result, you need to establish a suggestion at the Subconscious Mind and then reinforce it powerfully. To establish a suggestion, it must first be acceptable. When a suggestion is acceptable, it goes into the Subconscious Mind like a hot knife through butter.

What makes any suggestion acceptable is its relevance to the client's desires and internal experiences. Repeating suggestions that are based on the client's desired outcomes and insights will encourage change to occur more rapidly by reinforcing the truth of the suggestion. For example, you can suggest that the client is learning, growing, and changing through the healing process.

Relevance and revelations provide evidence to support the truth of the suggestion. The truer the suggestion is, the more acceptable it becomes. For example, how does the client know that change is occurring? Where has there been a shift toward a better thought or feeling? What did the client discover? What do they know now that they didn't know before? How much better do they feel now than when they first began?

The things a person says to themselves, in the privacy of their own Mind, are always going to carry more weight than anything you might say. Why not use it? Autosuggestion was developed at the beginning of the twentieth century by Émile Coué. It was Coué who coined the famous affirmation, "Every day, in every way, I'm getting better and better."

Coué recognized that suggestions don't last unless you reinforce them repeatedly. This is something we're already doing. It's called self-talk. Autosuggestion uses this by having the client give themselves a suggestion by speaking out loud. With each repetition of a suggestion, the strength of the concept or idea it suggests grows more powerful.

First, establish an acceptable suggestion. For example, "Notice how much better you feel (direct suggestion). Feel good?" (Verify the acceptability of the suggestion before continuing).

Second, instruct the client to say the suggestion out loud. For example, "Repeat after me: I feel better."

Third, add something to it. For example, "I'm allowed to feel better."

In this example, autosuggestion is used to incrementally increase the client's willingness to allow change. The first suggestion establishes a Subconscious Truth (i.e., "I feel better.") Repetition reinforces the strength of the suggestion while opening the door to an additional acceptable suggestion (i.e., "I'm allowed to feel better.")

Ditch the Script

You don't need a script. Because every problem is the result of a life experience, you won't find the answers the client is looking for in any script. The answers are within the Mind of the client. That's where you need to go to find your suggestions. If you use your intake strategically, you can uncover all the information you need to formulate powerful suggestions. As a result, you won't ever need a script.

As you guide the client through the healing process, all you need to do is keep good notes. You'll have everything you need to create suggestions that speak directly to the needs of the client. Make note of insights, understandings, realizations, and shifts in thinking, feeling, and behaving. You can use these things to formulate suggestions during your Session Wrap Up. Feed empowering concepts and ideas back to the client as direct suggestions. Better yet, use autosuggestion. Let the client tell themselves what they most need to hear.

The best suggestions will always come from the client because these are the ideas that have the most power for them. Sometimes a script can be useful. Sometimes you just know that you have the ideal script that's the perfect match for a particular client. In this case, by all means, use it. Use your scripts to supplement the suggestions that come from the client.

The goal is to emerge the client feeling really good about having made this decision to work with you. Get them feeling the feelings that go with having realized their goal. The feelings are what make it real. What's it like to be enjoying their most important benefit? That's their Big Bang Benefit. Then add a few suggestions for how the benefits continue to grow and expand as you continue working together. Keep the client's eyes on the prize. That's their Therapeutic Goal.

Summary

The purpose of your Session Worksheet is to support you in guiding a healing process. It gives you a place to keep the critical information you need during a session. Because it's all contained on a single sheet of paper, it's right there, at your fingertips, whenever you need it. This gives you an easy reference sheet with all the information you need to facilitate the healing process. The key information you need to refer to in every session includes:

- Therapeutic Goal
- Conditions for Change List
- Benefits of Change List
- Important relationships, past and present

- Quality of each relationship
- Insights that arise during sessions
- Evidence of change
- Forgiveness Work

Your Session Worksheet gives you an easy-reference sheet with all the information you need to create suggestions that connect the dots, reinforce positive change, increase positive expectancy, and encourage the Subconscious Mind to continue the healing.

When it comes time to wrap up your session, all you need to do is pull out your Session Worksheet and create suggestions that speak directly to the client's hopes and dreams. At the end of each session, all you need to do is do a review to reinforce the healing that has been initiated using the 3 Rs in the Wrap Up Review:

- Relevant
- Revelation
- Reinforce

Your Session Wrap Up should make whatever happened during the session relevant to the client's Therapeutic Goal, Conditions for Change, and Benefits of Change. It should conjure images of a brighter future and give the client an emotional experience of what it means to be successful.

The Therapeutic Goal reminds the client of their purpose for doing this work for you. This is where you're going. Because the client is at the center of the therapeutic process, no matter what is brought to light during a session, it's going to be relevant to the client's Therapeutic Goal.

The Conditions for Change reminds the client what needs to happen for them to be successful. This is how the client is going to get where they're going. During your Session Wrap Up, encourage the client to imagine doing the behaviors that will allow them to achieve their Therapeutic Goal.

The Benefits List reminds the client of the real reason the client is taking this journey with you. The rewards of change are always emotional. During your Session Wrap Up, encourage your client to imagine enjoying the rewards of having taken action to realize their Therapeutic Goal.

The best suggestions will always come from your client because these are the ideas that have the most power for them. At the end of the session, these are the things you want to reinforce over and over again. Compound them powerfully. They'll go into the Subconscious Mind like a hot knife through butter.

Bonus Alert! You can download a free PDF template of the Session Worksheet here: www.tribeofhealers.com/download-ditch-the-script-session-worksheet/

CHAPTER 10:
Set Up for the Next Session

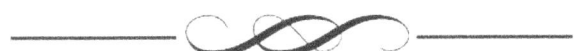

Regression Hypnotherapy is a journey of self-discovery and self-healing. During a regression session, there's a lot going on behind the scenes that you know nothing about. The Mind processes information a lot faster than a person can speak. As a result, not everything that's happening in a regression session is necessarily going to be shared with you. Clients can withhold information that might be relevant to their healing because they don't think it's important or are too embarrassed to tell you about it. They may not feel comfortable sharing it with you right away.

Realize that when the client emerges from hypnosis, they're still processing everything that happened in the session. Thoughts and feelings can be bubbling up to the surface of consciousness. Dedicating a few minutes to debriefing after a session allows the client to share thoughts, feelings, and insights that may not have been mentioned during the session. It also allows you to continue the healing work by reframing or reinforcing what's being shared to bring it into alignment with the client's Therapeutic Goal.

Between Sessions

Change doesn't happen during the session. It happens after the session. That's when post-hypnotic suggestions take effect. Because the healing process naturally stirs things up at a Subconscious level of Mind, the Subconscious Mind is going to continue to work on the client's issue following the session. It's going to be sorting through things and finding ways to integrate change. As this happens, the client may remember things that they haven't thought about in years. They may have interesting dreams. Uncomfortable emotions can bubble up to the surface, sometimes unexpectedly. The client needs to know that these things can happen and that they are relevant to their presenting issue.

The client needs to have realistic expectations. Healing is a process. Until the problem is completely resolved, the client will continue to be vulnerable to specific triggers in their daily lives. But you won't know what they are until you test the results between sessions. If something happens between sessions to trigger the client, or the client isn't able to hold onto the better feelings, this could actually be great news for you. But if the client is not prepared ahead of time, they could decide "hypnosis doesn't work." Nothing could be further from the truth. In fact, when the client bumps into an uncomfortable feeling between sessions, it's often because what you're doing *is* working!

Whatever happens between sessions tells you what the next step in the client's healing process needs to be. This is the information you need to uncover during the next session with the preliminary check-in. The preliminary check-in is a valuable part of a multi-session system because the only way you can ensure a complete resolution of the client's problem is to test the results between sessions. Your pre-hypnosis check-in gives you the information you need to guide the healing process effectively.

The following instructions are designed to set the client up to test the results between sessions. They form the basis of your preliminary check-in questions. In the client's first session, I always deliver these instructions just before emerging the client from hypnosis. I then repeat these instructions during the post-hypnosis debriefing to ensure that both the Conscious and Subconscious minds receive the instructions. In subsequent sessions, before sending the client out of your office, all you need to do is remind the client that one of three things can happen between sessions, and you'll be all set up for the next session.

Three Important Things

Between sessions, I want you to be very aware of your feelings because, following a session, three important things can happen.

First, you may feel better. That's good! That's what we want!

But you could also feel worse. The Subconscious Mind knows why we're doing this. It's going to be working behind the scenes between sessions. Sometimes, it can push stuff up to the surface because it wants this stuff healed. Just realize that it's part of the process. If you notice some uncomfortable feelings bubbling up to the surface, you let me know, and I'll take care of it, okay?

The third thing that can happen is that you may experience some ups and downs. That's normal. Everybody has ups and downs in life, right?

These instructions set the client up to expect something to happen between sessions. What's going to happen? Feelings. You want the client to pay attention to feelings. They should expect to be more aware of their feelings. Either they will feel better, worse, or have a few ups and downs, but you want them to be very aware of their feelings. That way, when they come in for the next session, you'll be all set up for the preliminary check-in.

Preliminary Check-In

Your preliminary check-in is simply a continuation of the client's previous session. The purpose of this check-in is to answer two important questions.

1. What do you remember about the last session?
2. What happened between sessions?

The first question is a way to pick up where you left off in the previous session. Instruct the client to mentally "do a little rewind" back to their last session with you. Then, ask, "What do you remember about that session?"

This question helps to refresh your memory. It can also be very revealing. Often, the client will have had some realizations after leaving the session. As a result, they will share more about that session than they did the first time. Giving the client a few moments to share in retrospect can result in more insights being brought to light. Insight is a precursor to understanding. Understanding is the Conscious Mind making sense of things, including why the client is taking this journey with you.

The second question is, "What happened between sessions?" Maybe the client slept better for the first time in ages. Maybe they noticed a reduction or even cessation of symptoms. On the other hand, maybe the client felt great following the session, but it only lasted for a couple of days. Maybe they lost the better feeling. Worse, maybe something happened to trigger them.

Better

If the client comes back and says they felt better following the session, you'll know that whatever you did in that session was effective. You made some headway. That's good. For example, if the client reports sleeping better, this is good news because many people are sleep-deprived. Just improving a person's sleep can make a big difference in how they think, and feel, and behave.

When the client reports any measure of improvement, what needs to happen next in their healing program is to celebrate success. Treat it like they just won the Olympic gold because the Subconscious Mind is qualitative, not quantitative. Reinforce every positive shift for the better before moving onto the next piece of the puzzle. This encourages the Subconscious Mind to continue to allow change to happen.

Worse

Even when the client feels great after they leave your office, they may not hold onto the better feeling. That's a clear sign that you haven't resolved the whole problem yet. That's fine. It just means there's more work to be done. If your client comes back and reports that they felt worse following the session, you'll know that you touched the "owie." That's where the pain of the problem is coming from.

The Subconscious Mind is letting the client know that it wants the problem resolved. This is great news! It also gives you the next step in the healing process. Focus on "that feeling." This is what their Subconscious Mind feels is most important. So, *that's* what you want to take care of next. The next logical step would then be to follow that feeling back to when it got started and resolve it there.

If the client got triggered between sessions, this gives you a recent event to work with. The next step in the healing process is to guide the client into hypnosis and return to the recent event. Review what happened and identify the specific emotion that got triggered. Follow "that feeling" back until you locate the ISE.

Ups & Downs

If the client reports experiencing some ups and downs between sessions, that's life. I like to say, "Welcome to Planet Earth." Ups and downs are a fact of life here on Planet Earth. What you need to find out is whether or not they got triggered. If so, what happened? What specific situation put them back on the emotional roller-coaster? This will give you a specific event to work with. That event has a specific set of feelings associated with it. This gives you a gateway to the past. Just bring up a feeling for a Bridge and go to work.

No matter what happens between sessions, as far as you're concerned, it's all good! It's simply information. You can use this information to help and guide you in facilitating the healing process effectively. Remember, if nothing changes, nothing changes. There's got to be some kind of movement following a session. You just need the client to notice that movement.

It only takes a couple of minutes following a session to prepare your client for the next session. Knowing what to watch for will help your client recognize when something is happening. This is the information you need to guide the healing process. Whatever happens, tells you what needs to happen next in the client's process.

CHAPTER 11:
Conclusion

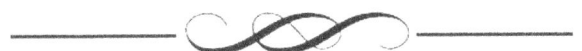

Do you want clients you can be successful with? Qualify your clients! It's unreasonable to expect to be all things to all people. You don't want to work with just anyone! You need clients that you can be successful with that are the right match for you and your level of qualification, experience, and skill. That's what will grow your knowledge, skill, and confidence. If you want to improve your results right away, use the Six Qualifying Questions to qualify your clients before booking them in for their first session.

Do you want to feel confident guiding a healing program? Get strategic with your intake process. Your intake process is much more than a brief conversation before guiding the client into hypnosis. It gives you a way to establish a Therapeutic Relationship with both the Conscious Mind and Subconscious Mind. Your intake can also be used to lay the foundation for establishing the Therapeutic Contract. While you take a history of the client's issue, you can be identifying the Symptom Pattern. You can be assessing the client's readiness to proceed with you. Used strategically, your intake gives you a preliminary uncovering tool that can provide the information you need to guide the healing process confidently and effectively. Use the ten Strategic Intake Questions to uncover the Symptom Resolution Keys.

Do you want to wrap up every session powerfully without ever needing a script? Create a Session Worksheet to support you while you guide the healing process. All the information you need to guide every healing session is right at your fingertips. And you can use it to wrap up your sessions powerfully—without ever needing a script.

To guide the healing process effectively, you need to establish a clearly defined Therapeutic Goal. This is the reason the client is taking this journey with you. The Conditions for Change provides the specific information you need to formulate targeted suggestions, establish milestones of change, create short-term coping strategies, and test the results. The Benefits of Change give you the client's motivating factor. You can use them to compound all the rewards of achieving the Therapeutic Goal.

Your Session Worksheet also helps you to keep track of additional insights, evidence of change, and Forgiveness Work as you continue to guide the healing process. At the end of each session, all you need to do is pull out your Session Worksheet and connect the dots with a Wrap Up Review.

Change doesn't happen during the session. Change happens between sessions. That's when post-hypnotic suggestions take effect. You won't know whether a change will last unless you test. Immediately after emerging your client, you can set up for the next session by reminding the client of Three Important Things that can happen between sessions. This sets you up to test the results between sessions. In the client's next session, you can pick up where you left off by using the two preliminary check-in questions. This sets you up to facilitate the client's next session.

So that's it.

I want to help you change how you think - about the hypnosis, the client, and the results—so you can grow a referral-based healing practice. That's the best kind.

Success is always going to be in your setup. You now have everything you need to ditch the script and set yourself (and your clients) up to be successful in your Regression Hypnotherapy sessions.

What's the Next Step?

The Devil's Therapy is a complete system comprised of a three-phase, seven-step protocol that will transform your hypnosis sessions into healing sessions that consistently deliver real and lasting results. Hypnosis to Healing is the second book in a series.

If you like what you've learned so far, please take a moment to write me a review. Your feedback helps others to decide whether this book is right for them.

If you are a teacher of Regression to Cause hypnosis, *The Devil's Therapy* can help to empower your students in their sessions with clients. As they gain experience, it will help to deepen their understanding of the healing process. As they shine in the work they do with clients, the light will reflect upon you.

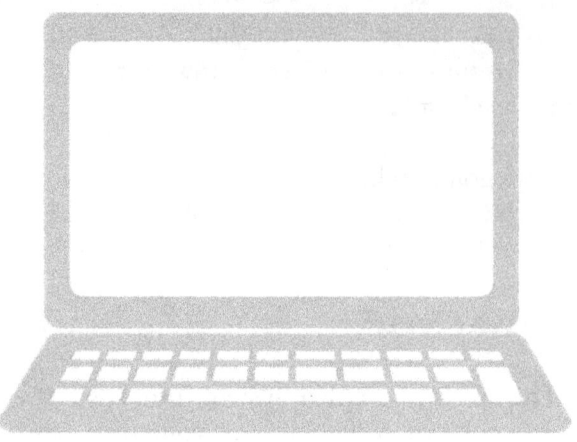

Ready to learn more?

Join the Tribe to receive weekly updates at www.tribeofhealers.com and get access to this awesome free course! **The Hypnosis Practice Business System Course** gives you an overview of how to grow a referral-based regression hypnotherapy practice in five simple steps.

You'll find a list of **recommended books and resources** here: www.tribeofhealers.com/wendie-recommends

On Facebook? Join the **Regression Hypnotherapy group**. That's where I hang out!

www.facebook.com/groups/32039528511828

Got questions? Post to the group or send me an email! I will reply. wendie@tribeofhealers.com

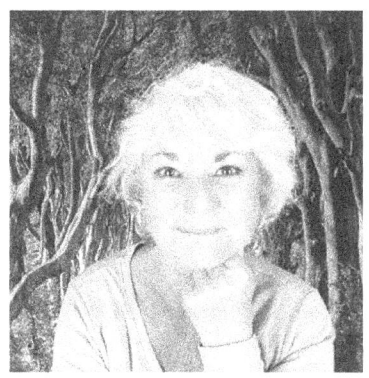

Wendie Webber

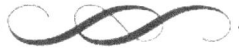

With over thirty years of experience as a healing practitioner, Wendie brings a broad range of skills to her unique approach to regression to cause hypnosis.

She is an Omni-Hypnosis graduate, 5-Path practitioner, Transactional hypnotherapist, Alchemical hypnotherapist, Satir Transformational Systemic therapist, and Regression Hypnotherapy Boot Camp participant.

Before hypnosis, Wendie owned a self-help bookstore where she explored spirituality, psychology, and energy-based healing.

Wendie is the recipient of the 2006 5-PATH Leadership Award and the 2019 Gerald F. Kein OMNI Award for Excellence in Hypnotism.

She enjoys an eclectic lifestyle on Vancouver Island, British Columbia, Canada, surrounded by nature, oracles, and cats. Her courses are available at TribeofHealers.com

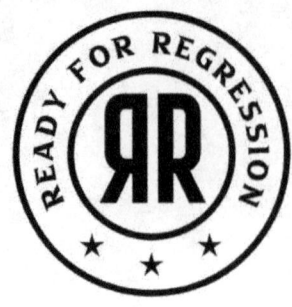

Get Ready for Regression!

Get immediate access to over 20-hours of step-by-step on-demand instruction in regression to cause therapeutic hypnosis.

Get clear. Get confident. Get ready!

The Ready for Regression First Session System Course is a proven 5-star rated system. Gain the confidence you need to guide your clients through the multiple healing processes of Regression to Cause Therapeutic Hypnosis.

> *IT WORKS!!!! I just finished a NEW session with a NEW client located in Asia. I had my semi-completed session manual with me that I put together based on your training course and . . . wow. It works. Confidence was back. Client felt great. Deep trance. I could go on forever. In short - thank you, Wendie. I put your course and method to real life and IT WORKS!!!!!! It works!!!! A huge suffocating hug to you!!! Thank you!!! And I didn't even complete all the courses yet!!!*
>
> *~ Jo Nontakorn*

Learn more at TribeofHealers.com (click the Courses tab)

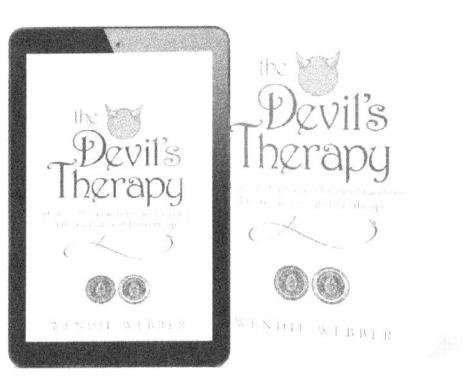

Get The Devil's Therapy: Hypnosis Practitioner's Essential Guide to Effective Regression Hypnotherapy

Discover how a **200-year-old fairy tale** reveals a complete system for facilitating effective regression hypnotherapy. Turn your hypnosis sessions into healing programs and get results that last. Learn the 3 essential phases of effective regression hypnotherapy hidden within a Grimm's Fairy Tale. Discover the "why" behind the "how-to" of regression to cause hypnosis.

Get clear. Get confident. Get results that last.

- Step-by-Step Guide for the Professional Regression Hypnosis Practitioner
- 3-Phase System to Achieve Lasting Results
- 4 Universal Healing Steps
- 7 Step Protocol to Transform Your Regression Hypnotherapy Practice

Available on Amazon. Learn more at: www.devilstherapy.com

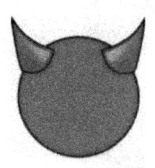

www.ingramcontent.com/pod-product-compliance
Lightning Source LLC
Chambersburg PA
CBHW020258030426
42336CB00010B/823